BEAUTIFUL
AWAKENING

Feel Your Best

Radiate Beauty

Experience Longevity

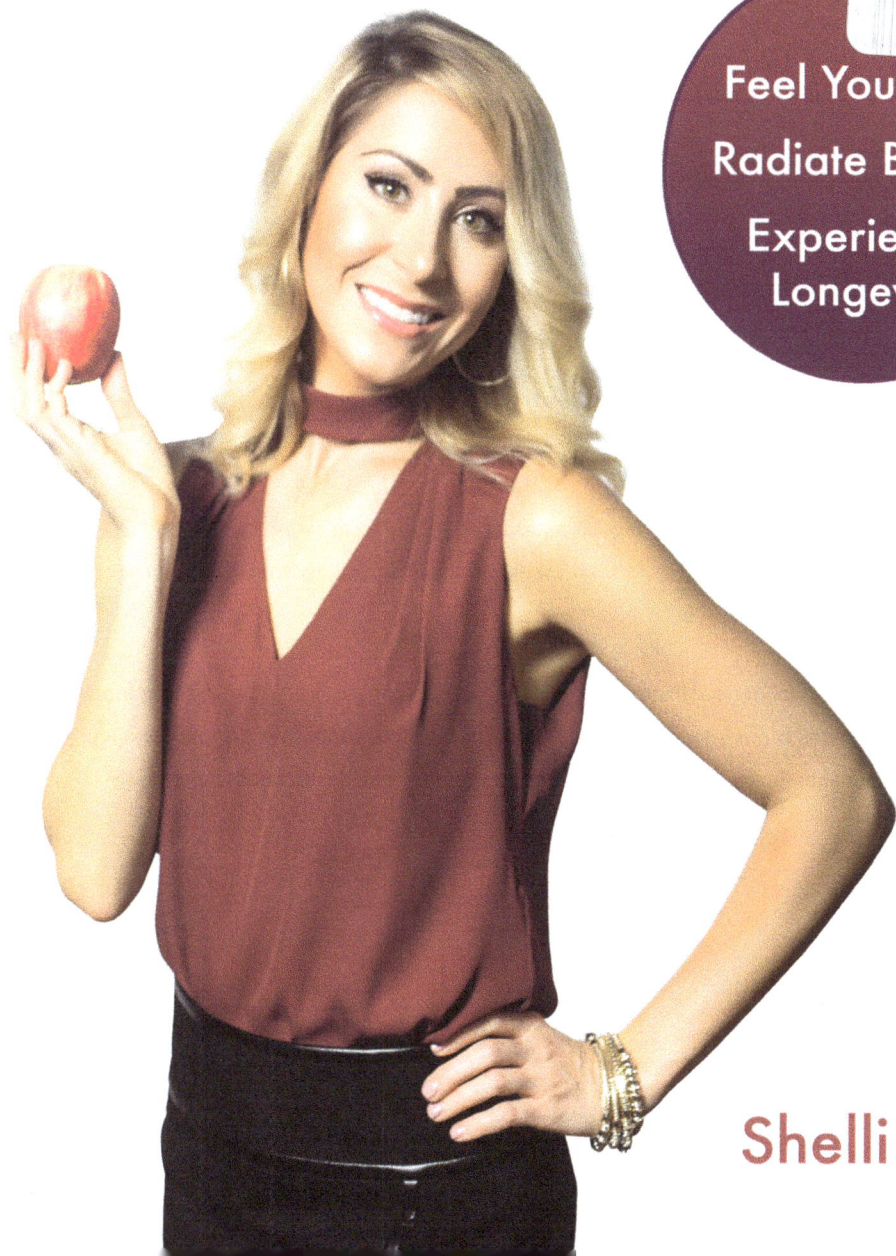

Shelli Belleci

Beautiful Awakening

Copyright © 2018 by Shelli Belleci

To contact the author, visit
www.ShelliBelleci.com

978-0-692-12518-2

Printed in the United States of America

FOREWORD

Beautiful Awakening is a book that is filled with knowledge and a step-wise approach to restoring your personal beauty with food. It can be the go-to bible for anyone wanting to start a plant-based journey. It is also a simple and quick start guide for someone looking at food as medicine, especially to heal from the inside out. The specific recipes you have here not only stimulate your taste buds but also enhance the beauty of the cells. It is very educational and scientific. The recipes are specially designed to help people restore their natural beauty, energy, and vigor while reducing inflammation and the need for infirmary. This book is packed with information, making every word important. You can finish this book in one sitting as it is written with such simplicity and logic that you acquire the education provided by the whole plant-based world in just this one book. Shelli's journey is authentic and very relatable for anyone struggling to stand apart due to personal choices, and will find sound advice here.

- Nisha Chellam - Medical & Holistic Dr.

DEDICATION

This book is dedicated to all the beautiful souls on this earth, including our animal friends. They, like us, have feelings, and many experience unnecessary pain and suffering daily. May this book help to positively change lives and spread a ripple effect that lessens torment and increases happiness, health, and joy. I would also like to dedicate this book to my daughter as a message that you can accomplish anything you put your mind to. Never let anyone or anything get in the way of letting your light shine. Thank you God, for giving me favor, wisdom, and strength.

ACKNOWLEDGEMENTS

Writing this book has been a project that requires attention and focus to help bring it to life. Many weekend nights were spent at my laptop both at home and in coffee shops all to produce, research, and work. Thank you to Nicole Barton, who took beautiful pictures of me and the recipes included in this book. I had so much fun at each photoshoot. Amie Olson, thank you for the incredible book design contributions, and Amanda Filippelli, for your editing magic.

Putting everything together took many hours and I could not have done it without friends near and far encouraging me along the way. I am also thankful to the health pioneers, authors, and doctors who have trekked out before me and provided education and knowledge about functional medicine, true health, raw foods, juicing and plant-based living. To my supporters, friends, family, and coworkers: I missed birthday parties, weddings, baby showers, and social events while I was working in my writing cave. I am deeply grateful for your belief in me and your understanding! I love you all.

TABLE OF CONTENTS

INTRODUCTION

As I look back on my life, I realize that my childhood and adolescent years shaped me to accept conventional ideologies about health and beauty. I grew up on the standard American diet, full of meat, dairy, sugar, and processed foods. Though my parents cooked many homemade meals, I still faced health challenges. Like many other American families, roasts, fried chicken, breaded meats, garlic bread, cheese, desserts, and pasta were among our standard meals. We also ate plenty of fish, bacon, burgers, and lunch meats. As a child, I remember questioning where the meat on my plate came from and I pondered whether I should eat meat or not.

Instinctively knowing that eating meat felt wrong to me, I experienced a deep and inherent compassion for animals. I think a lot of children feel this way. One night at dinner with my dad, we were having lamb, and I was probably six or seven at the time. I decided to ask him where the lamb came from. He told me the meat was the lamb, and I broke down into tears, shocked at the reality of what I was hearing. It is pretty common for children to react with shock, sadness, and disgust when they find out they are eating dead animals, or the characters they were reading about, like Babe or Nemo. I especially hated that idea. Despite my shock and concern, I ate what my family provided and had no major health problems until my later teenage years and early adult life.

The food in school was not the greatest, and that was all I ate for lunch. My junior high snack bar was filled with cookies, nachos, cinnamon rolls, and artificially flavored sugar "juices." I ate that junk every day for lunch, and rarely ate breakfast. In high school, vending machines sold soda, and students sold candy bars for fundraising. I often drank a Mountain Dew and ate a Snickers bar for breakfast. What a disaster! I spent all day eating empty calories. The truth is, many people start their days like this to the tune of doughnuts and sugary blended coffee drinks. Teenagers rarely care about nutrition and, at that age, it feels as if you'll live forever.

My first health hurdle came about when I was around seventeen years old. My doctor pre-scribed me birth control pills to "regulate" my hormones since there appeared to be a problem. A natural approach was not something discussed with me. I was told that my hormones were seriously imbalanced and I was at risk for polycystic ovarian syndrome. My doctor told me this could make it difficult for me to bear children later in life. Trusting the doctor's advice, I ended up taking the medication, thus consuming synthetic hormones for nearly seventeen years.

When I started the medication, I immediately gained twenty pounds. People might assume I would have been unhappy about that, however, it didn't bother me much at the time since I was tiny and had been underweight my whole life. Little did I know that I was teaching my body to rely on xeno hormones (a.k.a. "man-made") and running the risks of the unhealthy side effects of birth control consumption. Since these hormones are man-made, they are structured differently and are not used by our bodies in the same way as natural hormones. Relying on xeno hormones suppresses the body's natural ability to produce its own hormones and increases estrogen and insulin resistance. Numerous studies have found that birth control pills increase the risk of breast cancer (depending on the estrogen dosage) upwards of 60%. They also increase the risk of having a stroke.

Like most young women, I followed current fashion trends, idolized celebrities, obsessed over models, and read all the beauty magazines like a junkie. I aspired to be an actress one day. It wasn't long before I was on a mission to mold myself into the Hollywood ideal, and trying to look like that consumed me. I soon graduated high school and went off to college.

In the beginning, I was having the time of my life. I joined a popular campus sorority and socialized at party after party after party. I majored in psychology and took my studies seriously. I guess you could say I was well rounded. Drinking alcohol, coffee, and Diet Coke in more than moderate amounts became the norm for me. The party lifestyle was a lot of fun, but after a few years, I craved something different. I felt unfulfilled, empty, and depressed. I was ready to live a life of purpose and step into my authentic self as God created me to. I battled negative thoughts about myself and my life. I still do. I spent a lot of late nights either out at social events or studying for tests. It wasn't long before I put on an additional twenty pounds and took up smoking cigarettes. Self-awareness smacked me in the face one day, and I had to do something about it right away! So, I became bulimic, and lived in complete denial about it.

Everything looked good on the outside, but on the inside, I was dying. I was studying art and taking classes in subjects like nutrition, psychology, weight lifting, and ballet at the University of California Santa Barbara. My backyard was the Pacific Ocean, and it appeared that my life was pretty much a dream. I had decent grades and a lot of beautiful friends, yet I was completely disconnected from my true self. I felt spiritually void, and far from nature and peace. An awful feeling that I could never measure up plagued me, and I did not know how to accept and love myself.

The eating disorder became an unhealthy coping strategy as I struggled to process and control the world around me. I don't remember ever talking to anybody about things like body image, self-love, and eating disorders on a personal level, yet eating disorders are so common among young women and teens, especially in college. I was feeling a lot of pressure to maintain my school performance, and emotional issues were buried deep inside. Pressure to stay thin, beautiful, smart, and successful can drive a young woman to do just about anything, even destroy her health. My life felt out of control and I knew this unhealthy pattern was unsustainable. Intuitively, I felt there was something more outside the boundaries I was living in and this was my personal cry for help. Where was my direction in life? It was as if I was a caterpillar trapped inside a cocoon, dying to experience metamorphosis, to be a happy, healthy butterfly with beauty and magnetism, experiencing peace with myself and the world around me.

This went on for a few years, and it wasn't until the end of my senior year of college that I decided to take an alternative path. I took my health into my own hands and learned about veganism, juice fasting, and the raw food lifestyle. What I learned was so impactful and it changed my life forever! I educated myself as much as possible in these subjects and was fascinated to learn about how food and juicing could heal me in so many ways. I stumbled across some health books like *The Miracle of Fasting* by Paul and Patricia Bragg, *The Sun-Food Diet Success System* by David Wolfe, *Juice Fasting & Detoxification* by Steve Meyerowitz, *The Raw Food Detox Diet* by Natalia Rose, and more. I have these authors to thank for the information they published, which launched me on a journey to health, freedom, and increased happiness. I completed a few juice fasts, which were the most profound and clarifying experiences of my life at the time.

I was on an extreme roll. My friends and family were concerned with my dietary shifts. They were convinced I had an eating disorder. I laugh because when I had one, nobody said anything. It wasn't until I turned to eating fruits and vegetables to heal myself that anybody took notice. It's ironic that when people eat the worst foods on the planet, like white flour, meat, ice cream, and fast food, nobody has a problem with it. The second somebody refuses those foods for health reasons and starts exclusively eating fresh, whole foods, people become concerned, like there's something wrong with that.

I didn't care because I felt great and I knew I was doing the right things for myself! Like being born again, my true self was unleashed, and God had spoken to me in many ways. The days of binging, purging, cigarettes, alcohol, and Diet Coke were over. I finally discovered my true self, and I knew where I wanted to go in life. The things and people who were out of alignment with my future went their own ways, and I had finally stepped out of the box I felt trapped in for so long. Really, I was just following the crowd, trying to fit in, being a "good" daughter, and doing what other people wanted me to do. Where was my voice? I didn't have one, and I had to learn to be myself, love myself, and accept myself. I am still doing that.

The changes I made were not easy. At that time, raw foods and juicing were not mainstream or as popular as they are now. I had to completely rebuild my social network from the ground up. That was okay with me because, deep inside, I was rejecting mediocrity and the norm. Though I didn't realize it then, I was asking people to love me for who I was, not for who they wanted me to be. It's not always possible for so-called friends and family to be as understanding and accepting as you'd like them to be.

I still kept hearing that small voice inside my head, nudging me into a new direction, realizing the gifts God gave me. I was experiencing a beautiful awakening. Detoxing from old foods and relationships was tough because a lifetime of chemicals, medications, processed foods, emotions, and pesticides were all trying to escape my body, and it wasn't pretty. This is called a healing crisis. I pressed on and continued with my plant-based lifestyle because I felt great. Nevertheless, juicing and raw food veganism helped save my life and I am so glad I discovered and put into practice what I had learned back then.

I developed a passion for yoga and ballet and could not get enough of either. After college graduation, I studied a bit of ballet in Chicago and that was fun and adventurous. I moved back home after that trip, and the nastiest case of depression cast its shadow over my life. The darkness was debilitating. I felt helpless, hopeless, and without direction. I had slipped back into poor eating habits and, once again, I turned to raw foods and juices to get myself in the right state of health to do something about my life and future.

As a young twenty-something with big dreams to become an actress, singer and dancer, I shared these goals with a well-meaning family member. I was told those ideas were pie in the sky and I needed to get a "real job." This led me to believe I wasn't good enough to become successful, and the drift began. Nevertheless, I played it safe and I got my master's degree and a stable job. I was burying myself in even more of a mountain of student loan debt. I became a teacher to have a "real job" because that seemed like the logical thing to do. Sure, it's a good idea to have a back-up plan, but make sure that back-up plan is in alignment with where you envision yourself long-term. Always believe in yourself. And why garner insurmountable debt for a career you don't absolutely want with your heart and soul? Remember: the work you choose plays a big part in your health and quality of life. Choose it wisely.

While in graduate school, I went back and forth between eating meat and veganism. I also had my daughter and went through a divorce in less than five years. I let it take me down emotionally and mentally. I was faced with being a single mom who had taken close to a year off from a career in teaching to stay home and raise my child. I had to pick myself up and move forward with my life one day at a time. I was spent! I began to suffer from major digestive distress, anxiety, and had been diagnosed with acid reflux disease (a.k.a. GERD). I was drinking a lot of coffee once again and started using energy drinks and other stimulants to work, work out, pursue business, and be a super mom.

Slowly, my health was deteriorating. Doing this over time led to major burnout and a crazy case of adrenal fatigue. I remember laying down on my bed one night and literally feeling like I could not move. This was alarming and scary! Once again, I had to go back to ground zero, get myself back on track and in balance. The energy drinks were causing my heart to palpitate and that was the straw that broke the camel's back. You mess with your heart, you mess with your life. I was DONE, tired of feeling frazzled and tense, needing balance and grounding desperately. On top of that, I was spinning my wheels and not getting the results I wanted. What was a girl to do? You guessed it. Cut the crap and go back to raw foods, juices, veganism, yoga, and God. Have you noticed a pattern yet?

It was then that I learned about how gluten was damaging my health and I omitted it from my diet. I felt much better just by doing this, but not completely. Life went on, and I was still allowing stress to get me down, until I learned that stress is really just an excuse to feel bad. I did not have to let those things affect me, and neither do you. The greatest lesson I learned was to accept what I could not change and to act on the things I could. I decided to become a health coach and enrolled in the Institute for Integrative Nutrition health coach program. My life was coming together with even more alignment and I was thrilled.

I learned so much about health, lifestyle, nutrition, and I got connected with many amazing, like-minded people. It was worth it because my life would never be the same. I learned about meditation and started practicing breathing techniques. I also learned about how caffeine, wheat, dairy, gluten, and sugar were negatively affecting my health and beauty. Feeling like I had found myself again, I was thriving using nutrition and lifestyle techniques! My future was realigning with my destiny and I was healing.

I want to inspire people to discover themselves like I did and inspire them to live life alive and with power, true to their authentic selves. Life is too short to live it any other way, and you do not have to suffer with poor health, skin problems, depression, or anxiety. You also do not need to rely on medications to "fix" you.

I now allow myself to dream and take action. Doing this is empowering and fun. You can do this, too! My wish is that this book will inspire you to connect with your gifts. Becoming the best version of yourself is something you will never regret. We are always a work in progress, never finished, and self-development keeps us moving forward and looking ahead. The secrets to success are to find and connect with the right mentor (someone who does what you want to do and is getting results), never give up, and learn from your mistakes and adjust course when necessary. I certainly have learned a lot over the years.

To this day, I can safely say that I am off the diet hamster wheel, not counting calories or eating artificial sugar-free *this* or low carb *that*— "diet" foods made in labs, laden with chemicals. Eating fresh fruits, vegetables, nuts, and seeds allows me to eat as much as I want until I'm full without any concern about gaining weight or feeling guilty about food. This way of eating is not boring either, and it's not like you are limited to eating just salad all the time. Try some new recipes and learn raw food preparation techniques. I no longer suffer from digestive distress or acid reflux. My skin has improved dramatically, and I was able to stop taking all medications. In addition, I was also able to identify food intolerances that were robbing me of health, beauty, and happiness. I feel truly blessed for this journey and all I have in life. Raw foods and juicing has completely transformed my health. Eating a raw vegan diet shaves about ten years off your appearance and internal health, and it's no secret that diet, exercise, and self-love go a long way in that arena, too.

The truth here is that a plant-based lifestyle, exercise, and stress management works for everybody when done right. What you eat is your choice and perfection is not the goal. Everyone wants to feel great, look smashing, and feel empowered in their lives. Why wait any longer or stay stuck in the fear of experiencing something great, something epic, something life changing for yourself, the earth, and others? I believe in the saying, "Be the change you want to see in the world," and I hold that phrase dear to my heart. You will make a positive impact not only in your life, but in the lives of others.

If you are ready to begin this journey and see for yourself, then walk with me and let's get to it! Who taught you not to believe in yourself? Who told you that you aren't beautiful or that you're less than any other? Who put you down, hurt you physically or emotionally? Nobody who matters! Stand up for yourself and stand up against the bullies of the world. People who are hurting hurt others. Believe in yourself and your abilities. Defeat fear and lies head on with the truth that anything is possible, because you are stronger and more beautiful than you think. You will find when you are confident and when you believe in these concepts that plenty of others will align with you and follow suit. Make it a point to seek out people and network with those who value you and love you for who you are no matter what. In turn, be the person you need to others. You are beautiful, loved, and you deserve the best! Embark on this journey with me like today is the first day of the rest of your life. Marianne Williamson wrote some words that linger and motivate as they empower us to go after our true potential in this life. Here is what she wrote:

> Our deepest fear is not that we are inadequate. Our deepest fear is that we are powerful beyond measure. It is our light, not our darkness, that most frightens us. We ask ourselves, *Who am I to be brilliant, gorgeous, talented, and fabulous?* Actually, who are you NOT to be? Playing small doesn't serve the world. There is nothing enlightened about shrinking so that other people won't feel insecure around you. We are born to manifest the glory of the spirit that is within us, and as we let our own light shine, we actually unconsciously give other people permission to do the same. As we are liberated from our own fear, our presence automatically liberates others.

Let these words resonate within you and lift you up because they are truthful. After all, life is a gift; a completely valuable gift. We only have one life to live, and we live it day by day, moment by moment. All we have is now. Yesterday is gone, so let us not look back as we plan and envision the best future for ourselves. Tomorrow is only a concept, one to look forward to as we plan and live responsibly. Each present moment is what we do have, and the choices we make in each present moment define our quality of life, how we live, love, and thrive. I say make each moment count as much as possible, strive to love in each moment, and do not focus on that which does not serve you. Taking care of yourself allows you to better serve others. Have an open and giving heart. Love yourself and connect with God. Eat and move today, setting yourself up for how you want to feel tomorrow. Love like you're on borrowed time, and cherish this life with grace and gratitude, shining like the true star you are. I speak of love so much because it is a strong force, and it can tear down the walls of hate and fear. Being the essence of life, love gives life meaning and value.

With all of that said, take a moment to check in with how you are feeling at this very moment. Give yourself some space and sit upright comfortably. Close your eyes, take a deep breath, and go within. How do you feel? Are you happy, sad, tired, lonely, energetic, or feeling out of shape? Is your life so crowded by the needs of others that you have lost touch with how you feel and what you need? Focus your attention within your body. Starting from the top of your head, mentally scan down your body, and move your awareness all the way down to the bottom of your feet. Feel the weight of your body as you sit up in a comfortable position. Take some slow, deep breaths in and out. Now open your eyes. What did you learn about how you are feeling in this moment? Could you use more energy? Do you want to get into better shape or gain more confidence? What are you are doing to take care of yourself, and is what you are doing working? How is your digestion? Does what you eat agree with you and give you energy? How is your skin? Do you live to eat or eat to live?

Many people have high standards for their education, relationships, career, and finances. Often, health and fitness get put on the back burner when, really, wellness in these areas is the foundation for living a high quality of life. There are three pillars of strength in health: mental, physical, and spiritual. They all feed into one another and share equal importance. What you eat gives you energy and physical health that, in turn, induces a positive mentality, which is cultivated through intentional thinking and a spiritual connectedness. Feeling alive and having energy to do the things you love is important and not worth sacrificing for material things. After all, we cannot take possessions with us when we leave this earth, so it's in each moment we should allow ourselves joy as we journey through seasons in life.

What are your goals? Do you want to lose weight and keep it off, reverse aging, increase beauty, heal your digestive system, clear up skin issues, or have a renewed zest for life? Do you want to be more confident and connected to your authentic self and gifts? I challenge you to live passionately, not passively or miserably. You have everything you need right now to get started, and now is the time to start! By design, life is a concept in which we accept responsibility for our decisions, create a vision, set goals, and make choices aligned with what we aim to achieve. Change is always possible, no matter where you are starting from, and transformation is powerful. The truth is, you don't have to be on a diet forever, or go back and forth in numbers on a scale like a yo-yo. I dare you to throw away your scale. I did this years ago, and it helped me tremendously to focus on my specific health needs and the way my clothes fit rather than numbers on a scale.

Once we stop obsessing over what to eat and start living freely in our bodies, enjoying the pleasure of real food, other areas in our lives improve dramatically. Mental space becomes available and we can experience more clarity. All it takes is open mindedness as you discover and learn to adopt new and fresh ideas for looking and feeling your best. Fill your life with the right foods, activities, people, and experiences that leave no room for anything else that weighs you down.

CHAPTER 1
THE JOURNEY

Why I Choose Vegan

I remember when I was at the happiest place on earth. You guessed it. Disneyland! Since I was with my mom, daughter, young nephew, and sister, we had to eat at the happiest restaurant on earth. That place is Goofy's Kitchen at the Disneyland Hotel where the characters come out to dance and sing with you. The restaurant is buffet style and they bend over backwards to make sure your dietary needs are met. I thought, "What the heck, I'll have some cheese pizza on gluten-free crust." I mean, who doesn't love pizza?! This was a mistake.

The whole five minutes of pleasure from eating the pizza was not worth the month it would take to clear up the aftermath! I made a note to self: skip dairy. Cheese and ice cream were just not worth it anymore. I said goodbye to dairy products for good, and I was getting closer to health and freedom in my body. I honestly don't even miss them.

There I was, all gluten-free and dairy-free, like a diva. It was really beginning to feel as though I could only eat very specifically. Okay, but I was still experiencing a lot of digestive distress. Sometimes it felt better not to eat anything and just drink water. It felt like my whole digestive system was inflamed. As the days went on, the pains came in waves and it always occurred after I ate. The uncomfortable feeling left me stifled at times because it was difficult to speak or function with the discomfort. There were days I longed to be curled up in a ball somewhere until the episode passed. This was not okay, especially because it was happening while I was at work, in the process of managing a second-grade classroom. Imagine that. That's not fun for anybody.

It had been a long day of teaching, wrapped up in a long week of working and single parenting. I look back and remember many nights of eating dinner on the fly while helping my daughter with homework, cooking, cleaning, and working on side hustles. All this made me a bit delirious, and while grocery shopping a few days before, I picked up what I thought was a gluten-free vegan pizza. Well, it was vegan, but not gluten-free, and I clearly needed to avoid gluten at this point for digestive health. I had misread the box.

While I was busy multitasking and eating this pizza, little did I know what was about to happen later that night. I thought I was going to die! To make matters worse, I had jury duty the next day! I was in so much pain that I called my mom at 3 a.m. to let her know I might need her to take me to the hospital. Because of all this, you bet I am conscious about what goes in my mouth, and no, I'm not just trying to be a skinny bitch or a food snob. Nobody wants to feel that way and they shouldn't have to.

I knew that gluten and dairy were problematic because anytime I consumed them, whether deliberately or accidentally, I became sick and uncomfortable. But what else was going on? I had to get to the bottom of this. Symptoms like stomach pain, fatigue, bloating, brain fog, depression, and an inability to think clearly are all telltale signs of intolerance. Going back to the drawing table and looking for other causes of distress, I was beginning to take into consideration how food intolerances, caffeine, and stress were affecting my health. Though I was eating a healthy diet abundant in fruits and vegetables with small amounts of fish, chicken, soy and grains, I was still feeling sick, anxious, and rather miserable.

Food Intolerance or Allergy

The terms "food allergy" and "intolerance" are common today because of the healthy/green movement. A food allergy is different from an intolerance, and intolerances are quite common and due to pesticides, additives, chemicals, and genetically modified organisms. A true allergy is when the body treats a substance as an invader and produces white blood cells to fight off the intruder, which can include food, airborne substances, or chemical compounds. This abnormal reaction ends up doing more damage to the body than to the allergen. A food intolerance is when a specific food cannot be digested properly and adverse reactions occur such as gas, bloating, headaches, sleepiness, brain fog, or skin rashes and acne. These adverse reactions are not normal and should not be ignored. Nobody wants to deal with these things and they shouldn't have to. Once you are able to identify the food causing the reaction, the pleasure of not having the reaction will outweigh the desire of having the food itself. Some of the foods people are most intolerant to are wheat, dairy, soy, strawberries, shellfish, chocolate, eggs, tree nuts, and peanuts. Listen to your body. How do you feel when you consume these foods?

There are a few ways to pinpoint a food intolerance. If you have a true food allergy, you probably already know it, and it's best to talk with your doctor about your concerns. Food intolerances, on the other hand, can be difficult to diagnose and medical testing is not always accurate. If you suspect a food may be causing a problem, it is helpful to undergo a cleanse. This eliminates a list of foods and beverages from your diet for a period. After eliminating the food, you can reintroduce it in isolation and note if there is a reaction. Then, the food should be eliminated for another couple of weeks. If there is a reaction again, it is wise to eliminate it completely to feel your best.

Another method to pinpoint food intolerances is to rotate your foods. Eat a specific group of foods for four days and then switch to a different group and repeat the cycle. You can choose as many foods on a specific day as you like, but it is essential that no single type of food be ingested more often than every four days. Keep a food diary and write down everything you eat and drink in a day. Take notes about how you feel afterwards and for the next day or two. Sometimes a reaction does not occur until hours after consumption, the next day, or up to the next three days. I discovered my sensitivity to soy products this way. It's a misconception to think that you have to eat a lot of soy on a vegan diet. Remember that what is best for one person may not be best for another, so always listen to your body and discover what works best for you.

To pinpoint specifically which foods were the culprits for me, I eliminated all the possible offenders (gluten, dairy, grains, soy, sugar, caffeine, and alcohol) for a time. You may be thinking, *What is there left to eat?* Plenty! Trust me. Healing was brought forth into my life once again from eating only fresh raw whole foods, smoothies, and juices that could restore and rebuild my mind, body, and soul. After going raw for a few months, my skin improved, I looked younger, and my hormones balanced themselves out! My digestive problems were a thing of the past and I didn't feel any food remorse. I never have to count calories or worry about portion control. I simply eat when I'm hungry and stop when I'm full. I knew I could always revert back to this way of eating to feel better whenever I needed to. That is what I did once again, and I see no need to turn back!

I continued to dig deeper into my specific health problems and solutions. Diet wasn't the only solution, and the idea of integrated health dawned on me. Is conventional medicine treating people with integrated health techniques? If you have a headache, we have been taught to take Tylenol. If you are breaking out, we have been told that diet is not the problem and are prescribed medications and topical creams. The body is made up of systems and organs that work together cohesively. When one is out of balance, other systems of the body are affected. We must look at our systems this way and treat them to bring the body into balance as opposed to covering symptoms with medications. Because I was experiencing breakouts, I had to investigate why that was happening. I discovered the role the liver plays in eliminating toxins from the body, and when it cannot do so properly, toxins will eliminate in other ways (through headaches and through the skin for example).

Knowledge is power, and power without action is useless. What good does it do to know what is good for you and neglect to do the things that would bring health, happiness, and freedom? I follow a high raw vegan diet as a rule of thumb and find that it brings me the best results. My health has improved dramatically and I feel better than ever! Nothing about this lifestyle feels difficult or restrictive because this is my choice and based what is best for me. Once you discover the delicious alternatives and try more recipes, you may find that you do not miss other foods. Over time, the good feelings, energy, and beauty you experience will surely outweigh the old miserable feelings that came from eating the wrong foods.

You have the choice to discover what works best for you and there's no need to live with any dietary labels. Whether you choose to be vegan, vegetarian, pescatarian, or a carnivore, that's your choice. You could be flexitarian, meaning you consciously eat what works to support your health day by day. I choose vegan because it's best for the animals and the environment. Plus, I look and feel better eating that way. I care enough about animal welfare to feel right at home with excluding animal products.

Eat like you care, because every time you make a purchase, you are voting with your dollars for what you support. Know that, without a doubt, we were made for wonderful things, and that health is much like any other journey in life. It takes time to heal, get to the root of your health issues, prevent problems, and build up strength and immunity. Taking a pill to fix your health problems only masks illness, as if you are telling your body you don't want to listen to its needs and address them. It is your birthright to be healthy and so worth the attention and effort you give into taking care of yourself one day at a time. Being healthy all starts with the plate.

CHAPTER 2

AUTOIMMUNITY

Were you thinking whole grains are healthy foods? They are, but not for everybody all the time. If you suffer from autoimmune disease, your immune system is compromised and damages its own normal tissues as if something is wrong. In this case, grains could be robbing you of the health you deserve and causing inflammation in your body. Autoimmune disease affects tens of millions of Americans alone and is linked to more than eighty diseases. There is a spectrum of autoimmunity within which a person may experience symptoms measurable based on a scale. By going through the following questionnaire created by autoimmune disease specialist Dr. Amy Meyers, you can start to measure whether or not you have an autoimmune disorder as well as its severity. The good news is there is a protocol to follow to bring about healing.

You must heal your gut. A healthy gut revolves around the premise of gut permeability, and a healthy gut serves to break down foods and absorb nutrients. In addition, our gut produces serotonin, and when gut health is bad, anxiety and depression can occur due to low serotonin levels. Skin health, hormonal balance, toxin/waste elimination, and energy production are all related to gut health. Leaky gut syndrome associated with autoimmune disorders is a controversial phenomenon that is in the early phases of research. The lining of the gut becomes damaged and undigested food, bacteria, and waste leaks into the bloodstream. Gluten is known to contribute to leaky gut syndrome and this causes inflammation and sickness.

Some traditional medical practices do not seem to recognize leaky gut syndrome as a medical disorder due to the lack of scientific data and clinical trials to back up its diagnosis and treatment. Specializing in treating autoimmune disease, Dr. Amy Meyers teaches how to control inflammation in the body with her developed protocol. There are various issues involved with autoimmunity such as small intestine bacterial overgrowth, food sensitivities, candida, parasites, and low stomach acid. Here, I will provide you with the questionnaire developed by Dr. Meyers to track autoimmune symptoms. Assess your symptoms over the past week and rate them on a scale of 0-4 based on how strong any symptom is occurring.

0 = none 1 = Some 2 = Mild 3 = Moderate 4 = Severe

Head	Ears	Lungs	Digestion
____headaches ____migraines ____faintness ____trouble sleeping Total _____	____itchy ears ____earaches, infections ____ear drainage ____ringing ears, hearing loss Total_____	____chest congestion ____asthma, bronchitis ____shortness of breath ____difficulty breathing Total _____	____nausea, vomiting ____diarrhea ____constipation ____bloating ____belching, gas, heart burn, indigestion ____intestinal/stomach pain/cramps Total_____
Mind	**Mouth, Throat**	**Skin**	**Emotions**
____brain fog ____poor memory ____impaired coordina-tion ____difficulty breathing ____difficulty deciding ____slurred/stuttered speech ____learning/attention deficit Total_____	____chronic cough ____frequent throat clearing ____sore throat ____swollen lips ____canker sores Total_____	____acne ____hives, eczema, dry skin ____hair loss ____hot flashes ____excessive sweating Total_____	____anxiety ____depression ____mood swings ____nervousness ____irritability Total_____
Eyes	**Heart**	**Weight**	**Energy, Activity**
____swollen, red eyelids ____dark circles ____puffy eyes ____poor vision ____watery itchy eyes Total_____	____irregular heartbeat ____rapid heartbeat ____chest pain Total_____	____inability to lose weight ____food cravings ____excess weight ____insufficient weight ____compulsive eating ____water retention, swelling Total_____	____fatigue ____lethargy ____hyperactivity ____restlessness Total_____

Nose	Joints, Muscles	Other	
_____nasal congestion _____excessive mucus _____stuffy/runny nose _____sinus problems _____frequent sneezing Total _____	_____joint pain/aches _____arthritis _____muscle stiffness _____muscle pain/aches _____weakness, tired- 　　ness Total _____	_____frequent illness/ 　　infections _____frequent/ 　　urgent urination _____genital itch, dis- 　　charge _____anal itch Total_____	**Grand Total:** _____

Next, add up the total from the questionnaire, and then answer the following questions:

Your total from the questionnaire: _____

1. Based on your symptoms related to the questionnaire, do you think you have an autoimmune disease? If yes, add 8 points. _____

2. Do you have more than one autoimmune disease symptom? If yes, add 10 points. _____

3. Do you have any diagnosis ending with "itis" such as arthritis, colitis, pancreatitis, sinusitis, or diverticulitis? If yes, add 10 points. _____

4. Do you have a first-degree relative (a parent or sibling) with an autoimmune disease? If yes, add 10 points for the first relative and two points for each additional relative. _____

5. Do you have a second-degree relative (a grandparent, aunt, or uncle) with an autoimmune disease? If yes, add 5 points. _____

6. Are you a female? If yes, add 5 points. _____

Your total from the questions above: _____

Add your total from these questions to the questionnaire total for a complete total. The following numbers will tell you your place on the autoimmune spectrum.

Your complete total: _____

Less than 5	5-9	10-19	20-39	40-79	Greater than 80

If your total is 5 or less, then your inflammation is very low and you are not at risk for developing an autoimmune condition. If your total is 5-9, you have small risks for developing an autoimmune condition, however, you could still benefit from eating an anti-inflammatory diet (the same goes for when you are not at risk). If your total is from 10-30, you are at mild to moderate risk for developing an autoimmune condition and are experiencing significant inflammation. Following an autoimmune protocol for healing is your best bet to avoid an autoimmune condition. If your complete total is over 30, you are at moderate risk due to heredity, high levels of inflammation, or you have already developed an autoimmune disorder.[1]

Inflammation is the root cause of so many symptoms. It is wise to pay attention to where you may fall on the spectrum. The good news is that we are all bio-individuals, meaning that what works for one person may or may not work for the next. At the end of the day, you must listen to your body and experiment with foods to see what best supports your health and energy levels. If you suspect grains are negatively impacting your health, start by assessing your symptoms with the questionnaire provided in this book, and then eliminate grains for a period. Next, add them back into your diet one at a time to see how you feel afterwards. If you have any abdominal pain, fatigue, brain fog, headaches, or other symptoms after reintroducing the grains, then you should avoid eating them.

I would only recommend omitting grains if you fall significantly on the autoimmunity spectrum. Omitting beans and legumes are also beneficial for people who experience digestive distress and/or inflammatory symptoms. Sprouting and soaking raw seeds and legumes increase their nutritive qualities and digestibility. I recommend doing this if you want to eat them, especially if you are vegan or vegetarian, to get more protein into your diet. Nuts are a good source of protein but are listed as something to avoid if dealing with autoimmunity. I was experiencing autoimmune symp-

---

1   Amy Meyers M.D., *The Autoimmune Solution, Prevent and Reverse the Full Spectrum of Inflammatory Symptoms and Diseases,* 2015, Harper Collins.

toms but have found that by eating raw-vegan, I can tolerate nuts and sprouted legumes in moderate amounts. I soak them when I can and eat them with greens. Grains, nuts, seeds, and legumes are staples for many people on a vegan or plant-based diet and are great foods.

As with any health condition, we must be vigilant and take responsibility for our own health and wellbeing, so always listen to your body. It speaks to us through emotions and physical feelings via pain. Begin to examine your emotions and feelings and think, *Where is this coming from?* Always communicate with your doctor as needed for concerns about serious medical conditions at large. Something you can do right away to address any health or beauty discomfort is to juice fast. This is an age-old remedy for many ailments as it works to remove what is possibly offending the system and allows for healing and the removal of toxins. Reintroducing clean plant-based whole foods after a fast allows you to discover which foods best serve your body.

CHAPTER 3
GUT HEALTH AND RESTORATION

Hippocrates said, "All disease begins in the gut." It's safe to say you are *not* what you eat, rather you are what you digest. Digestion is the process of assimilating food into energy by absorbing vital nutrients through the small intestine before elimination through the colon. Health, the gut, and intestinal issues are related. SIBO (small intestinal bacterial overgrowth), candidiasis, leaky gut syndrome, and irritable bowel syndrome are some of the challenges people face around gut health. It all boils down to intestinal health and healing the gut. So how does someone achieve this?

When I started learning about digestion and gut health in an effort to help myself, I learned that restoring the gut takes care of many challenges. If you are having any sort of gastrointestinal issues, one of the first steps to helping yourself is to get to the root of your problem. This can be confusing because many conditions have overlapping symptoms. There are some important things to consider when healing your gut. In my journey, I further assessed my diet, colon health, food combinations, stress, and psychology. I believe a lot of my failing digestion was brought on by stress and food, so I went to work on both. According to the National Institute of Diabetes, Digestive and Kidney Disease, nearly 60-70 million people are affected by digestive diseases. These diseases account for 21.7 million hospitalizations, 245,921 deaths, and $97.8 billion in direct medical costs. The diseases responsible for these striking numbers include chronic constipation, diverticular disease, abdominal wall hernia, gastroesophageal reflux disease, gastrointestinal infections, hemorrhoids, inflammatory bowel disease, Celiac Disease, and non-celiac gluten sensitivity.[2] These statistics are mind blowing and certainly present an economic strain to have such enormous medical costs associated with this epidemic.

Candidiasis was something I came across during my quest to heal, and I noticed many of the symptoms for candida overlap with symptoms of autoimmunity and gut related issues. Like everything else, I dove right into how we address candida with diet. Candida is a fungal infection in the body caused by yeast overgrowth and can affect health in a variety of different ways. Some

---

2   National Institute of Diabetes and Digestive and Kidney Disease, (2014). Digestive Disease Statistics for the United States. Retrieved from https://www.niddk.nih.gov/health-information/health-statistics/digestive-diseases

of the symptoms associated with candida that I was experiencing were depression, sleep problems, irritability, mental fogginess, anxiety, dizziness, attention deficit, obsessive compulsive tendencies, and an irregular heartbeat. Once I began to nourish my body (gut lining) with key nutrients from raw fruits, vegetables, juices, smoothies, and fermented foods rich in probiotics (while avoiding dairy and grains), I began feeling better than ever.

Because negative emotions can also contribute to a compromised gut, it is important to reflect on your own emotions in relation to your health issues. Stress may be affecting your body's ability to digest and function properly, because people often experience a gut-brain phenomenon in which prolonged psychological or environmental stress induces illness in the body. This is what happened to me. The nervous system in the gut is sometimes referred to as a "second brain" because it relies on the same types of neurons and neurotransmitters that are found in the central nervous system (brain and spinal cord). After sensing that food has entered the gut, neurons lining the digestive tract signal muscle cells to initiate a series of intestinal contractions that propel the food farther along, breaking it down into nutrients and waste.[3] When the nervous system is affected by stress, digestion is slowed or stopped to focus the internal energy on the problem. That is exactly what happened to me when my digestion was at its worst. I was allowing my work environment to perpetuate the whole thing. I also noticed that anytime I experienced relational stress, I would experience similar digestive distress. It wasn't until I started following a regimen of fresh fruits and vegetables, smoothies, and juices that I got my digestive issues under control and the pain I felt in my gut disappeared.

Digestion, beauty, and energy are connected, and this relationship begins with the premise that digestion is meant to be sound and regular. This means everything we eat and drink becomes processed with ease and we are free of disease, illness, and suffering. You will have the most beauty and energy by addressing your colon or gut health. If you are suffering or have suffered from digestive distress, you know that living with it can miserably hinder your quality of life, like it did mine. If you have not experienced digestive distress, perhaps you have had problems with constipation. If you have, you know how much happier you would feel to be free from that forever.

There are different factors affecting digestion, and if you have problems, it is important to get to the root cause of them right away. Some issues that may hinder digestion are worth considering, like gluten intolerance, celiac disease, autoimmune disorders, dairy intolerance, colon congestion, a need for body detoxification and cleansing, irritable bowel syndrome, overeating, environmen-

3   Harvard Mental Health Letter, Harvard Health Publishing. August 2010. Stress and the Sensitive Gut. Retrieved from www.health. harvard.edu/newsletter_article/stress-and-the-sensitive-gut

tal stress, and/or psychological stress. These problems stem from an unhealthy gut. Think of the gut as an environment, a microbiome. Technically speaking, there are millions of live bacteria and other organisms working together symbiotically doing their jobs within that microbiome. When the gut environment gets off kilter, things start to deteriorate and fall out of whack.

Healthy gut lining has small intestine surface cells that fit tightly together, but when these cells become damaged, gaps occur between the cells and food particles can slip through, causing a host of other problems. This is known as leaky gut syndrome. Functional medicine teaches that once the microbiota in the gut is healed, you should be able to eat otherwise noted healthy foods again. This is great news, however, people might develop a fear of eating specific foods due to an association with past pain and suffering after consuming those foods. This why I love whole plant foods. With peace of mind, I know that what I eat will not cause me pain and that is priceless. I can eat raw fruits, vegetables, nuts, seeds, and sprouts as much as I want, and my digestive woes are behind me.

What About Grains?

There is a notable amount of controversy in the diet world—enough to make your head spin. Many doctors and health experts will recommend eating whole grains, soy, and legumes as part of a healthy diet, and others will say to avoid these foods. In my opinion, neither side is right or wrong because nutritional needs entirely depend on each person and their lifestyle. A person might be reactive to certain foods depending on the amount of stress they are experiencing at that time while also being non-reactive under times of ease and flow. I am not saying that grains are bad or that they should be avoided by everyone. If you can eat them and you feel great, that is awesome!

I have found tremendous healing benefits from excluding not only gluten from my diet but grains as well. This was the final step that has taken my healing to the next level. Once I did this, my digestive problems improved dramatically, my blood sugar stabilized, unexplained mental fog and fatigue diminished, and my skin improved. If you can relate to my story in any way, try going grain-free and see if you feel better. There are amazing grain-free recipes out there for nearly every traditional savory dish and sweet dessert created by mankind. Once you learn what the alternatives are, it's easy as pie to eat that way.

If you choose to eat grains, here is a tip. Soak them before cooking. This makes them more digestible so you can add them as a healthy part of a well-rounded and balanced vegan diet. Eating grains like brown rice, millet, and oatmeal are good choices, especially for those just starting out with plant-based eating. For others, it's better to shy away from the grains for some time to control inflammation.

Inflammation is linked to many conditions like acne, eczema, IBS, arthritis, fibromyalgia, heart disease and cancer. Grains can cause an inflammatory response in the body due to specific proteins or anti-nutrients called lectins and phytates. These plant toxins bind to cell membranes, making them nutritionally unavailable. Phytates and lectins are present in legumes, soy, seeds, barley, wheat, rice, beans, and nuts. They create inflammation while blocking nutrients from vitamins and minerals, thus wreaking havoc on your health. In plants, lectins evolved to provide a protective barrier, so seeds can pass through animal digestive systems and be dispersed. Therefore, people have trouble digesting lectins, and raw soaked kidney beans are even poisonous due to lectin content.

By soaking grains for twenty-four hours and rinsing them often, lectins and phytates are reduced and rinsed away. Proper cooking techniques also do away with the harm posed by these antinutrients. The popular paleo diet has convinced many to forego grains and legumes. This diet shuns all grains, beans, and soy, focusing primarily on meats, fruits, vegetables, and nuts. Despite what we know about whole grains being good for us, we need to keep an open mind to heal. Soaking, cooking, and sprouting grains and legumes makes them more digestible, and these techniques are worth experimenting with. If you have any of the afore-mentioned issues, consider avoiding grains and legumes for an amount of time to bring about gut healing. As I always say, have nuts, seeds, legumes, and grains in moderation for optimal digestion.

Gluten or No Gluten? That Is the Question

I got a call from my aunt one day informing me that a relative of ours has celiac disease and a cousin of mine was so sick from a compromised digestive system that she could only eat blended foods and drink them from a straw. I could relate to that as I felt that way a lot. She also told me her entire family, including her grandchildren, were gene carriers for celiac disease and were going gluten-free as a preventative measure. My aunt, cousins, and grandmother all boasted about how they were feeling better than ever as a result. "Yikes," I thought. This is something relevant to me. I questioned my own gluten tolerance, which then caused me to learn more about the topic, which led me to question grains.

Gluten is a substance made up of two proteins present in cereal grains, especially wheat, which is responsible for the elastic texture of dough. Gluten intolerance is an inability to process gluten in the body, and a person with this issue would experience negative side effects after eating it. Celiac disease is a serious autoimmune condition that can occur in genetically predisposed people where the ingestion of gluten leads to damage in the small intestine. It is estimated to affect 1 in 100 people worldwide. If you carry the celiac gene, celiac disease can develop at any time from something that triggers it (food and medicine especially).

Some of the symptoms of celiac disease include bloating, gas, abdominal pain, joint pain, irritability, diarrhea, constipation, delayed growth, itchy skin rash, poor digestion, weight gain, significant and unexplained weight loss, missed menstrual periods, discolored teeth or loss of tooth enamel, tingling or numbness in hands and feet, fractures or thin bones, canker sores, infertility, depression, bipolar disorder, type 1 diabetes, and more. Keratosis pilaris, known as dry skin on the back of the arms with little red bumps could be related to a Vitamin A and or fatty acid deficiency because of malabsorption or inflammation. For those who are Celiac or gluten sensitive, intestinal villi are damaged and flattened, after gluten consumption and nutrients are not absorbed properly. Problems occur, such as eczema, which is another skin issue that can be associated with gluten intolerance.[4] The most common skin disturbance associated with gluten is atopic dermatitis, aka eczema. This could be due to a food intolerance or allergy to the gluten itself. Many dermatologists dismiss the idea that food is related to skin problems, however studies suggest that people with non-Celiac gluten sensitivity notably improved in their conditions after adopting a gluten free diet.[5] Personally, I have noticed improvements in my skin, digestion, cognition and moods after going gluten free. It is worth trying out to alleviate symptoms.

I saw how my symptoms aligned with many of the gluten related symptoms I had researched. I had never even heard of the disease before, let alone ever considered that healthy foods such as wheat and other whole grains were ruining my health. In my opinion, it is wise to avoid gluten whether you are intolerant or not. I think it's difficult to digest and linked to inflammation and bloat-

4   Burkhart, A. February 2017. Gluten Causes Keratosis Pilaris (a.k.a. "Chicken Skin"): Fact or Myth? Retrieved from http://theceliacmd.com/2016/02/gluten-and-keratosis-pilaris-chicken-skin/
5   Bonciolini, V., Bianchi, B., Del Bianco, E., Verdelli, A., & Caproni, M. (2015). Cutaneous Manifestations of Non-Celiac Gluten Sensitivity: Clinical Histological and Immunopathological Features. Nutrients, 7(9), 7798–7805. http://doi.org/10.3390/nu7095368

ing in general. Most people who have celiac disease are not even aware that they have it, and gluten is linked to many disorders. If you are avoiding bread, beer, gluten filled desserts, and grains that are going to cause you to feel inflamed and bloated, you will thank yourself for not eating them. Be aware that there is a right way and a wrong way to go sans gluten. What many people do not realize is that gluten is not just present in wheat, barley, and rye products. All grains have some form of gluten in them, although some are considered gluten-free and safe for people with celiac disease (like rice and amaranth).

Gluten has become a hot topic in the health arena for a variety of reasons. By now, you have most likely either dismissed having any problem with it or are still not sure what the big deal with gluten is in the first place. Perhaps you have decided to omit it from your diet because it's trendy. Maybe you laugh at the gluten debacle and scoff at all the hype. Have you taken the time to investigate the research and problems associated with gluten and how it may be negatively impacting your beauty and health? You still may be feeling confused, so let's keep this simple. Stay away from processed foods and junk. Stick to organic whole foods and cook at home as much as possible. There is gluten in so many foods except fruits, vegetables, meat, nuts, legumes, and seeds.

The origin of the gluten grain is of significance because not all gluten is created equal. There are a few ways to discern if you should avoid gluten or not. One way is to omit it for some time, reintroduce it slowly, and note any changes in how you feel. Aside from true celiac disease, a large percentage of gluten-free followers are concerned with gluten intolerance. Traditional blood testing for celiac is accurate but could render a false negative result. You must be eating gluten when tested and intestinal biopsy is known as the gold standard in testing. Biopsy is invasive and a small percentage of people (1-3%) develop celiac disease. Stool testing is also an option for genetic testing. Even if you have the genes for celiac, like 20-30% of the population, this is not a guarantee you will ever develop the disease.

People are aware that there is an association between gluten and health. Even small amounts of gluten can cause a reaction for those sensitive to it. About 80% of celiac cases go undiagnosed, and people suffer without making the connection.[6] Even people without celiac or non-celiac gluten sensitivity can benefit from avoiding gluten containing foods for good reasons.

Today's wheat crops are hybridized in efforts to make them bacteria resistant. This is a dif-

6   Rubio-Tapia, A., Ludvigsson, J.F., Bratner, T.L., Murray, J.A., Everhart, J.E. *The prevalence of celiac disease in the United States.* The American Journal of Gastroenterology. 2012 October.107(10):1538-1544; quiz 1537, 1545. PMID 22850429

ferent and problematic wheat, unlike what our grandparents had years ago. Hybridization has formed new strains of proteins our bodies do not recognize. As a result, our bodies have not evolved to tolerate these proteins and respond as if a foreign invader has attacked. Our food is changing faster than our bodies ability to respond. Technically speaking, additives derived from gluten sneak their way into processed foods without anybody even knowing it. These are more reasons to prepare whole foods, unpackaged, and unprocessed at home as much as possible. You can control what goes into your food, and it tastes better, too.

Consuming gluten can cause a person with celiac disease to become extremely ill with a host of health problems stemming from flattened villi in the intestine. This makes it impossible for nutrients to be absorbed properly and contributes to leaky gut syndrome. This can cause more problems such as anxiety, depression, brain fog, bloating, constipation, weight loss, diarrhea, irregular periods, frequent colds, flu, infections, joint pain, excess weight, vitamin and mineral deficiencies, acne, eczema, and rosacea to name a mouthful. Sometimes, however, damage occurs in the body asymptomatically, and you might not be aware of the damage occurring internally.

Many commercial gluten-free foods are processed and have added sugar (many times with higher amounts of simple carbohydrates) than their gluten counterparts. There are a lot of gluten-free junk food choices on the market, and it's easy to think that by replacing traditional foods with a gluten-free alternative that your health problems will disappear. This is not true. Sugar is sugar, and refined carbohydrates are unlikely to ever really be on your side. Foods like gluten-free breads, crackers, cakes, and cookies made with refined rice and potato starch and other grain flours are best left to be consumed in moderation or avoided all together. The best way to lose weight on a gluten-free diet is with whole, natural foods and beverages. Gluten is present in many products like soy sauce, BBQ sauces, gravies, toothpaste, cosmetics, skin care, Play-Doh, shampoos, conditioners, medications, and more. In order for a product to be labeled as gluten-free, it must contain less than twenty parts per million (ppm), which is a really small amount.[7]

I like to avoid all products containing gluten besides food because I have noticed how sensitive my body is to even minute amounts. Overall, I feel better and avoid itchy rashes and breakouts by choosing gluten-free and natural shampoos, soaps, lotions, deodorants, and makeup whenever possible. This may sound daunting, but I have discovered products I love from cruelty-free companies and I feel great about my purchases. People who have celiac disease or are very sensitive should avoid

7   U.S. Food and Drug Administration, Questions and Answers: Gluten-Free Food Labeling Final Rule. (2017). Retrieved from https://www.fda.gov/Food/GuidanceRegulation/GuidanceDocumentsRegulatoryInformation/Allergens/ucm362880.htm

products that contain gluten, even though you might think it's too small to make a difference. I know what you are thinking. It seems like there is something wrong with everything concerning food and product choices these days. Once you cut through all the garbage, deciding what to buy becomes easy because it's quite simple. Simple, natural, and cruelty-free products are what you want to use.

All grains contain some form of gluten. Therefore, eliminating them from your diet is helpful for people suffering from inflammation. There are plenty of delicious options and recipes out there to fulfill every craving and dietary need you have. Going gluten-free is a surefire way to prevent inflammation, and that offers peace of mind. If you suspect you have celiac disease, be sure to contact a doctor with expertise and credibility in that arena. What it all boils down to is giving up gluten could lead you to a better quality of life and you don't have to give up the doughnuts. Gluten-free vegan doughnuts can be whipped up and they are delicious!

Fruit is the most easily digested of all foods and it passes through the digestive system quickly. Fruit is an ideal food loaded with its own enzymes. It can be considered a pre-digested (perfect) food. Eating fruit alone, or in mono meals, helps the body have more energy, the best digestion, and increased beauty. A mono meal means you are eating one type of fruit for a meal in a large enough amount to qualify as a meal. Eating mono fruit meals helps clear the colon of congestion and keeps your face looking fresh. For example, you could eat half a watermelon, five to seven mangos, or a large, satisfying smoothie with frozen bananas for breakfast or lunch. Not only is fruit great for digestion, but fruit is loaded with beauty vitamins, minerals, and antioxidants that slow and reverse the aging process. The digestive process requires a large amount of energy, and this is one of the reasons why people feel tired after a heavy meal. After a fruit meal, this is not the case. You may start to crave sunshine and exercise when consuming raw fruits and vegetables as your meals.

As age increases, the body's ability to produce digestive enzymes decreases. These digestive enzymes break down foods into carbohydrates, proteins, and fats (the building blocks for our bodies to utilize). Each enzyme is there to break down a specific food type, so if you are having trouble with digestion, it is important to follow food combining principles. Companies sell digestive aids made of fruit enzymes, such as papain (derived from papaya) or bromelain (derived from pineapple) to assist in digesting foods. These digestive enzyme products are perfect for people who experience gas or bloating after eating large amounts of raw fruits and vegetables. If this happens to you, don't worry and don't hesitate to eat fruits and vegetables or large salads.

If you are gassy and bloated after eating fruits and vegetables, then follow food combining principles and do some colon cleansing with enemas or colonics. The bloat and gas will go away once your colon and digestive system are cleansed and strengthened. The problem is not the fruits and veggies. The problem is a toxic colon that needs cleansing. Enzymatic supplements are also helpful if you are eating foods that are more difficult to digest, like animal proteins and grains, and especially when transitioning into a plant-based/vegan lifestyle.

These types of meals are rewarding in so many ways. Not only are they easier to digest, which maximizes nutritional absorption, energy and elimination, but they are easy to prepare and require minimal effort once you get the hang of it. Breakfast is a good place to start when adding in more raw foods to your diet. Ask yourself while grocery shopping, *What fruit sounds good right now? Mangos, melons, pineapple?* Purchase the fruits and vegetables that appeal to you the most and try to get mostly in season produce. Shop the fresh and in season produce at the farmer's market. It tastes the best! Stock up on those foods, eat from home, and refuse to visit the drive-through. Fruit is the best fast food. You grab it and go!

Smoothies are perfect to have as easily digested meals that bring vibrant health and beauty. The key is to have a significant amount of the smoothie to ensure you're getting enough calories. You can always boost your smoothie with plant-based protein, coconut butter, nut butter, maca powder, fresh greens, green powders, chia and hemp seeds for added satiety and energy.

Another way to increase digestion is to chew your food. Becoming aware of thoroughly chewing your food creates a mindfulness that may prevent overeating as well. It is a way of slowing down the process of eating and creating consciousness within the experience. I would say thirty to fifty times is a good start. I understand that nobody really counts how many times they chew their food. The point is that the more you chew, the better. Pay attention to the taste and texture of the food and how that changes after a time of chewing. Remember, the less work your digestive system must do, the more energy you will have. In turn, the body will focus its energy to heal and cleanse internally.

Heavy, improperly combined meals take the longest to digest and zap the body of vitality, energy, and beauty. Fruits and vegetables are high in fiber and water, which act like a broom to the digestive system, sweeping away what is not serving the body from the colon and moving things out. This is good because elimination should be happening anywhere from one to three times daily. If that is not the case, then increase your water intake, eat more raw fruits and vegetables, juices, smoothies, and consider getting colon hydrotherapy. Crowd out meat, dairy, and anything lacking fiber (like eggs). Improper elimination can also contribute to weight gain. If the colon gets backed up, then matter begins to putrefy. Toxins in the colon will look for other channels of elimination such as the skin and thus breakouts occur. The skin is a large eliminative organ. A juice fast is a great way to reset everything. When digestion is efficient and healthy, gas and bloating is not an issue.

There are different ways to go about cleansing, and entire books are written about colon health alone. Having a healthy colon is quite powerful, and it feels great to have optimum digestion. With high rates of colon cancer in America, colon health is an important topic people need education about. Many diseases manifest in the colon. According to the American Cancer Society, Colorectal cancer is the third most diagnosed cancer, and the third leading cause of death, with expectations to kill 50,630 people in 2018.[8] That's 50,630 mothers, fathers, grandparents, sisters, brothers and loved ones we don't want to lose! Plant-based whole foods are filled with fiber and help sweep through the colon, thus preventing cancer. Meat and dairy have no fiber and large amounts of them could cause problems. Think about a fast food meal of a burger, fries and a milkshake (loaded with sodium, saturated fat, and devoid of fiber, vitamins and minerals). Those types of meals do not move through the colon efficiently, nor do they nourish the body. Therefore, such food contributes to an unhealthy colon, obesity, and high blood pressure. Colon health is important to maintain when looking to maximize your health and beauty goals. Colon cleansing with diet, colonics, and herbs can reverse negative conditions associated with a toxic colon. Probiotics are what we call "good bacteria" and can be consumed for optimum nutrient absorption and digestion. They make a difference and help your body absorb minerals and assist in the elimination of toxins. With a healthy colon, all the vitamins and minerals from the beautiful fruits and vegetables you eat will come shining through from the inside and you will look amazing.

8   The American Cancer Society. (2018). Key Statistics for Colorectal Cancer. Retrieved from https://www.cancer.org/cancer/colon-rectal-cancer/about/key-statistics.html

CHAPTER 4

INSIDE OUT BEAUTY

Aesthetically, society deems a beautiful person as having clear, firm, glowing skin, bright eyes, and a head of full, glossy hair. Many people all over the globe spend countless dollars on facial creams, products, and other costly procedures to have clear, glowing skin. How many advertisements have you seen for skin regimens, chemical peels, medications, and laser treatments all with the goal to give people healthy, clear skin? We hear of using pills, creams, and costly procedures to improve skin conditions. We are told that food does not affect acne. I beg to differ! Eating more fruits and vegetables increases nutrition in the body, and this provides vitamins and minerals for beautiful hair, lean muscles, strong nails, and glowing skin.

Hormonal imbalances affect acne and, therefore, birth control pills often help to keep skin clear. I was prescribed birth control pills as a young woman to control hormonal issues, until seventeen years later when I became educated about the problems with them. Aside from that, I thought something must give, because I couldn't take those pills forever. Anytime I attempted to stop taking them, my hormones went crazy and my skin would break out, so not wanting to deal with that kept me going back to the pharmacy to fill my order.

As I approached my mid-thirties, I felt ready to let my body balance itself naturally and was willing to address the root issue at hand no matter what. I had to address my lifestyle habits, like sleep and stress, and take some effective herbal supplements. It took about two years for my body to readjust while on a vegan diet, but it did, and I am grateful to not have to rely on those pills any longer. About a year into that journey, I transitioned to a raw vegan diet (high raw) and that made a world of a positive difference. My period is regular for the first time ever in my whole life! Too much information, but ladies, it can be done. Yes, food does make a difference!

Think about it for a moment. Does it make sense that consuming fat, sugar, processed and low fiber foods would ultimately lead to a system that is out of balance, inflamed, and toxic? Not having beautiful, clear skin can really damage one's self-esteem and is an indicator that something is internally out of balance either physiologically, hormonally, or emotionally. Many beauty products such as cosmetics, sunscreens, fragrances, and other personal care products contain questionable ingredients that are toxic, carcinogenic, and endocrine disrupting. A great resource to learn more about safe cosmetic and personal care products is ewg.org.

Years back, when I worked in the makeup department at a high-end department store, I discovered and used some of the fanciest, most expensive skin care products on the market. I was surprised to find that they didn't perform any miracles on my skin. I feel like I would have been just as well off using over-the-counter drug store products. Finding and using the right skin care products are important, but it is far more important to invest in your beauty by cleansing the body, getting enough rest, managing stress, exercising regularly, and eating foods rich in vitamins, minerals, and antioxidants. You will see great results from doing this and an increase in your beauty. The following chart[9] lists foods, their health and beauty nutrient sources, and benefits. Include these foods into your diet regularly, and if some are unfamiliar to you, now is a great time to give them a try.

Beauty Foods

Food	Nutrient Source		Benefits	
Avocados	• Biotin • Potassium • Copper • Iron	• Vitamins A,C,E,K • Glutathione • Glutamine	• Anti-aging: protects skin from environmental damage	• Smooth, supple, youthful skin • Antioxidants • Anti-aging
Acai	• High in antioxidants • Vitamin C • B vitamins	• Omega fatty acids • Vitamin E • Fiber • Potassium • Calcium	• Anti-aging	• Brightens & renews dull skin
Almonds	• Vitamin E • Zinc • Calcium • Iron • Potassium • B vitamins	• Manganese • Selenium • Copper • Folate • Amino acids	• Protects against skin damage • Aids skin issues like psoriasis • Energizes • Vitality	• Nourishes dry hair & skin • Smooth, supple skin
Arugula	• High in vitamin A	• Vitamin C, K, iron, calcium, & fiber	• Protects skin from free radical damage	• Anti-acne

---

9   Kimberly Snyder, C.N., *The Beauty Detox Foods,* 2013, Harlequin Books.

Food	Nutrient Source		Benefits	
Asparagus	• Vitamin K: helps body to absorb calcium		• Detoxifying: prevents urinary tract infections & kidney stones	• Balances electrolytes • Reduces puffiness & bloating
Apples	• Vit A, C, K, • Calcium • Potassium		• Stabilizes blood sugar • Binds with & removes toxic metals • Clear, bright eyes	• Lowers cholesterol • Decreases risk of stroke and cardiovascular disease
Bananas	• Vitamin B6: reducing insomnia & irritability, promotes good digestion	• Magnesium: better sleep • Vitamin A - prevents constipation	• Essential amino acid tryptophan fights depression	• Potassium: satisfies sweet cravings • Moisturizes skin
Beets	• Iron • Calcium • Antioxidants • Magnesium	• Folate • Vitamins A,C,E • Alkaline	• Stimulates liver function • Oxygenates the blood	• Builds blood • Removes toxins • Brightens eyes • Anti-cancer
Blueberries	• Vitamins A,C,E • Selenium • Zinc	• Phosphorus • B-vitamins • Copper • Iron	• Low glycemic • Highest in antioxidants next to acai berries	• Strengthens eyes • Beautiful skin
Cabbage	• Vitamin A,C, E • Calcium • Magnesium • Potassium • B vitamins	• Iodine: assists thyroid & endocrine glands • Sulfur: heals wounds	• Minimizes deep lines in the face	• Boosts energy & muscle development
Carrots	• Calcium • Potassium • Iron • Fiber • Vitamins B1, B2, B6, C, K	• Biotin & vitamin A: shiny moisturized hair	• Anti-aging	• Keeps the scalp healthy for hair growth

Food	Nutrient Source		Benefits	
Celery	• Organic alkaline minerals: calcium, magnesium, potassium	• Potassium & sodium flush out fluids	• Calms the nervous system • Natural laxative • Lowers blood pressure • Supports kidneys & liver • Diuretic	• Decreases puffy eyes • Anti-inflammatory • Eliminates waste/toxins = increased beauty
Chlorella	• 50% protein • Contains all essential amino acids		• Cleanses digestive tract • Top detoxifier • Carries oxygen throughout the body • Fights candidiasis	• Healthy skin • Weight loss • Energy • Muscle strength • Alkalinizes/balances body pH levels
Cilantro	• Vitamin A, K • Calcium • Potassium • Folate		• Eliminates mercury from the body (from heavy seafood consumption)	• Less colds and flu associated with heavy metal intoxication
Coconuts/ Young Coconuts	• Iron • Potassium • Magnesium	• Calcium • High amounts of electrolytes	• Cellular cleansing • Regulates blood pressure	• Promotes youthfulness • Anti-aging
Cucumbers	• B vitamins • Potassium • Calcium • Iron • Magnesium	• Vitamin C • Enzymes • Silica	• Prevents bloating • Flushes kidneys • Anti-inflammatory	• Creates beautiful skin • Hydrating
Collard Greens	• Alkaline • Magnesium • Calcium	• Chlorophyll • Vitamins A, K, B1, B2, B6, & E	• Addresses and prevents dark under eye circles	• Brightens skin tone • Eases stress

Food	Nutrient Source		Benefits	
Chia Seeds	• Omega 3, 6 • Protein • Calcium • Potassium		• Lean/strong body • Keeps you full • Stabilizes blood sugar • Steady energy supplier	• Workout food stamina & endurance • Replaces amino acids post workout
Dulse	• Vitamins B6, B12, E, A • Iron • Zinc	• Calcium • Potassium • Magnesium • Iodin	• Iodine for thyroid health	• Minerals for growing & nourishing hair
Figs	• Vit A • Calcium • Potassium • Magnesium • Folate		• Heightens your inner glow • Clears colon of mucus which blocks skin nutrient absorption	Assists in blood cleansing Clears colon of toxins provides a laxative effect
Flax Seeds	• B6 • Calcium • Magnesium • Omega-3 fatty acids	• Folate • Iron • Zinc • Manganese	• Anti-inflammatory • High fiber stabilize fiber	• Healthy smooth nourished skin
Garlic	• Contains allicin Powerful germ annihilator		• Purifies blood & lymphatic system • Detoxifies waste • Clear skin • Deters yeast infections	• Digestive aid • Antiseptic • Anti-inflammatory • Stimulates the digestive tract • Assists with candidiasis

Food	Nutrient Source		Benefits	
Ginger	• B vitamins		• Stimulates collagen for firm skin • Anti-inflamma-tory • Antioxidant • Tightens & brightens skin • Stimulates digestion	• Improves digestion • Fights infec-tions • Increase hair growth • Lowers blood sugar
Hemp Seeds	• All 9 essential amino acids	• Protein • 3,6,9 omega fatty acids	• Builds long, lean muscle tone	• Vibrant skin • Hair • Nails
Irish Sea Moss	• Potassium • Chloride: dis-solves phlegm & inflammation	• Contains ionic minerals	• Soothes diges-tive tract • Helps respirato-ry problems • Wrinkles • Eczema • Thyroid func-tion • Fatigue	• Antimicrobial • Antiviral • Gets rid of infections • Skin mask • Dark circles • Sunburn • Hair skin & nails
Kale	• Free form ami-no acids • Vitamins A, C, E • Vitamin K • High in antioxi-dants	• Manganese • Iron • Copper • Calcium • Omega-3 fatty acids	• Fights cancer • Battles stiff joints	• Balances hor-mones
Lemon	• High in vitamin C		• Aids digestion • Flushes bacte-ria and toxins • Helps main-tain long term weight loss	• Fights wrinkles • Glowing, clear skin • Brightening • Alkalinizing
Nutritional Yeast	• Amino acids • B vitamins • Zinc • Selenium	• Magnesium • Manganese • Copper	• 3 tablespoons equals 9 grams of complete protein	• Strong, healthy hair

Food	Nutrient Source		Benefits	
Onions	• Vitamin A, C, • Sulfur • Calcium • Potassium • Iron • Silicon		• Strengthens capillaries protecting against varicose veins • Cleanse liver and skin	• Clear skin • Blood cleansers • Clears sinuses & digestive tract
Parsley	• Vitamins A, C,E	• Folate • Iron	• Detoxifier • Diuretic • Aids digestion • Blood cleanser Anti-cellulite • Creates that glow	• Prevents bloating • Flushes kidneys
Pears	• Vitamin C & E • B vitamins • Vitamin K • Copper • Manganese • Potassium	• Magnesium • Selenium • Calcium • Zinc • Folate • Iron	• Colon cleansing	• Removes toxins that age the skin
Papaya	• Enzyme papain	• Vitamins A & C	• Promotes digestion • Oxygenates the body • Soothes digestive tract • Healthy skin • Anti-wrinkle	• Repairs skin • Cleanses internally • Allows for nutrient absorption • Beautiful eyes • Gorgeous hair
Pineapple	• Vitamin C • Manganese: regulates blood sugar levels	• Bromelain: enzyme for digestion, breaks down protein	• Reduces inflammation & swelling • Cleanses blood • Improves circulation • Reduces mucus	• Reduces gas • Softens face • Anti-wrinkle • Anti-bloating • Develops collagen: firms skin • Soft gorgeous skin

Food	Nutrient Source		Benefits	
Pumpkin Seeds	• Zinc • Sulfur • Protein • Magnesium • Iron	• Vitamins A, C, E, & K • Phosphorus • B vitamins • Biotin	• Helps acne • Essential fatty acids for skin and scalp	• Strong & healthy hair
Radishes	• Vitamin C • Sulfur • Silicon		• Dissolves mucus • Allows nutrient absorption	• Cleansers & detoxifiers • Hair strengthening • Clean body = healthy hair
Red Bell Peppers	• Silicon	• High in vitamin C	• Repairs & regenerates collagen for firming the skin	• Supple, youthful skin
Sauerkraut Kimchi Fermented Vegetables	• B vitamins • Stacked with probiotics	• Vitamin C helps vitamin K synthetization	• Keeps yeast & fungus down • Strengthens immune system • Prevents constipation	• Eradicates food allergies • Beautiful clear skin • Intestinal health • Prevents intestinal infections
Romaine Lettuce	• Nutrient rich • Vitamin C • Beta carotene • Manganese • Vitamin B1, B2	• Iron • Chromium • Molybdenum • Vitamin K	• Builds blood	• Anti-aging • Eliminates free radicals
Sesame Seeds	• High in calcium • Iron • Zinc • Fiber	• Magnesium • Manganese • Copper • B complex vitamins	• Supports collagen & elastin • Anti-inflammatory	• Strengthens bones, joints, blood vessels

Food	Nutrient Source		Benefits	
Spinach	• Beta-carotene • Phytonutrients • Flavonoids • Vitamin A • Vitamin K • Folate • Selenium	• Manganese • Iron • Calcium • Magnesium • Zinc • Amino acids	• Prevents wrinkles • Youthful skin	• Anti-aging • Moisture retention
Spirulina	• B complex, D, K		• 60 % protein-easily absorbed • Increases stamina • Curbs hunger • Cleanses heavy metals • Reduces bad cholesterol • 10x the concentration of beta carotene found in carrots	• Ideal for athletes • Balances hormones • Optimizes cleansing and digestion • Boosts immunity • Prevents heart problems
Sprouts	• Calcium • Sulfur • Amino acids • Fatty acids	• Antioxidants • B complex • Iron	• Promotes cellular regeneration • Cleansing • Nourishing	• Predigested food • Easily assimilated nutrients
Sweet Potatoes	• Vitamin A, C, E • Biotin • B2 • B6	• Iron • Potassium • Manganese • Folate	• Stabilizes blood sugar • Protects against cancer & heart disease	• Skin brightening • Anti-inflammatory

Food	Nutrient Source		Benefits	
Raw unpasteur-ized Apple Cider Vinegar	• Potassium • Trace minerals		• Digestive aid • Antiviral anti-bacterial • Antifungal • Stimulates metabolism • Weight loss & fat burning	• Clears acne • Cures constipa-tion • Alleviates sugar cravings • Promotes growth of pro-biotics • Addresses candida & yeast issues
Turmeric	• Iron • Magnesium • Calcium • Potassium		• Anti-Inflamma-tory • Anti-cancer effects • Glowing, sup-ple skin	• Increased blood flow & cleansing • Prevents acne & skin disorders
Walnuts	• High in ome-ga-3 fatty acids • High in protein Vitamin E • Fiber • B vitamins	• Magnesium • Calcium • Potassium • Amino acid L-arginine	• Heals collagen & tissue • Increases anti-oxidant activity	• Contain mela-tonin, contrib-uting to good sleep
Watercress	• Calcium • Iodine	• Vitamins A, C, E	• Cleanses & oxy-genates tissues	• Glowing skin • Good for acne & eczema

If you have a problem with inflammation, depression, acne, or digestive distress, then it is your body signaling that there is a problem at large, and it must not be treated only as an isolative problem. Rather you must take your entire lifestyle into consideration.

When you feel better, you automatically look better. Think about all aspects of life when addressing a problem. With acne, diet is important, but stress management and emotional and hormonal health are equally important. Taking time to rest, fostering healthy relationships, and engaging in spirituality and self-love are all a part of the circle of life that contributes to overall health and beauty. If a person is eating healthy but not sleeping enough, dealing with toxic relationships, or debilitating work stress, then this can throw the system off balance. Eating anti-inflammatory foods high in water and fiber with a low glycemic load are the best foods for healing skin conditions. Also, making sure to not consume foods your body is allergic or sensitive to is a BIG piece of the puzzle. A diet high in fiber, whole, nutrient dense plant foods promotes a system of healthy organs working together in unity to provide clear, healthy skin. Each person is individual and that is why lifestyle must be curated to fit each unique person in a way that will support their needs.

The body is made up of seven major eliminative organs and the skin is the largest. When toxins are not eliminated properly by an unhealthy colon or a toxic liver, one theory is that the toxins will be eliminated through the skin. Sugar, coffee, and alcohol are all addictive substances and contribute to toxicity, which leads to breakouts if overly consumed. Cut these offenders out for thirty days and watch how amazing your skin looks. Does this mean that you should ban them forever? The answer is up to you, but it's not necessary to give everything up entirely. It depends on your lifestyle, goals, and struggles. For some people, complete abstinence from addictive substances serves them, whereas, for others, occasional indulgences are doable. Many of the longest living people around the world regularly drink wine, eat meat and seafood, and socialize, which feeds the relational need we have to connect with others and to have fun. Other groups known for longevity, like the Seventh Day Adventists in Southern California, completely abstain from alcohol and meat and also live long, healthy lives.

As you eliminate dietary offenders and get to a place where you are experiencing better health, you can certainly enjoy whatever it is you want in moderation. When I was suffering from what my doctor recognized as acid reflux, I had to eliminate some of my favorite foods and beverages from my diet for six weeks or any time the acid reflux became problematic. These were foods like chocolate, pineapple, coffee, and oranges. Once my acid reflux was under control, and my body became alkaline with the right foods, I could enjoy those foods again in moderation. If the symptoms you were having come back, you should know how to treat them and ask yourself if it is worth it for you to have those reactions and decide what other support you need.

Rock Your World with Food Combining Strategies

This is a life changer! By following certain food combining strategies, I became svelte, gained more energy, and greatly improved my digestion. It is simple once you get the hang of it. Properly combining food allows for more optimal digestion and elimination. Foods eaten in an optimal combination will be digested more efficiently and will not get backed up in your system. Improperly combined meals can clog up the system and takes longer to digest. When the body does not have to produce extra enzymes to digest improperly combined food, those reserves contribute to preserve youth in the body. Your skin will glow, your hair will shine, the whites of your eyes will brighten, your skin will be firmer and tighter, and you will have more energy to do all the things to live a healthy life. This includes work you love, time with family and friends, and exercise.

The practice of proper food combining is of great help to those who want more energy and/or suffer from digestive distress. The idea behind this is to not mix different food groups together (carbohydrates, fruits, and proteins) in meals. Each food group has a specific enzyme that breaks it down, and mixing certain food groups hinders digestion because the enzymes clash with each other.

Protease is the enzyme that breaks down protein into amino acids. Amylase is the enzyme that breaks down starch into sugar, and lipase is the enzyme that breaks down fats into fatty acids. For the best digestion, proteins are best paired with low starch vegetables. Carbohydrate rich foods like rice and pasta are best mixed with vegetables alone. One would not mix protein with carbs together in a meal (such as chicken and pasta) because this would impair digestion and require differing enzymes to break down the different food types. Fats are okay to combine with carbohydrates and proteins separately. For example, a large salad with greens, avocado, olives, and sweet potatoes would be a good combination. Another example is a kale salad with protein (sprouted nuts or legumes), plenty of raw vegetables, and avocado. Fruit should be eaten alone on an empty stomach, especially melons. If you are eating a high raw diet, you may find yourself able to break some of these rules because your body is not dealing with the taxation of cooked foods, dairy products, and animal products. I often add fruits like mangoes, apples, and pears to my green salads. Lettuce combines well with fruits and fats. Refrain from eating fruit at the end of a meal as this causes gas and bloating.

Included here is a guideline for plant-based food combining. It is good to know about food combining principles in general and to experiment, figuring out what is going to work best for you in terms of digestion. If you are vegan or vegetarian and do not suffer from digestive distress, then I recommend eating food that makes you feel good despite the rules. If combinations like beans and rice cause you problems, you could eat beans with salad, salsa, steamed vegetables and avocado, or replace the beans with rice instead. Do not worry about portion control so much because the idea is to eat until satiated, not stuffed. If you need a few helpings, go for it, but don't overdo it. Overeating causes digestive distress as well, and a good rule of thumb is to eat until you are 80% full. This may take some practice for those of us who love to eat! The good news is the damage will be minimal! Check out this food combining chart to help you create the most digestible beauty meals.

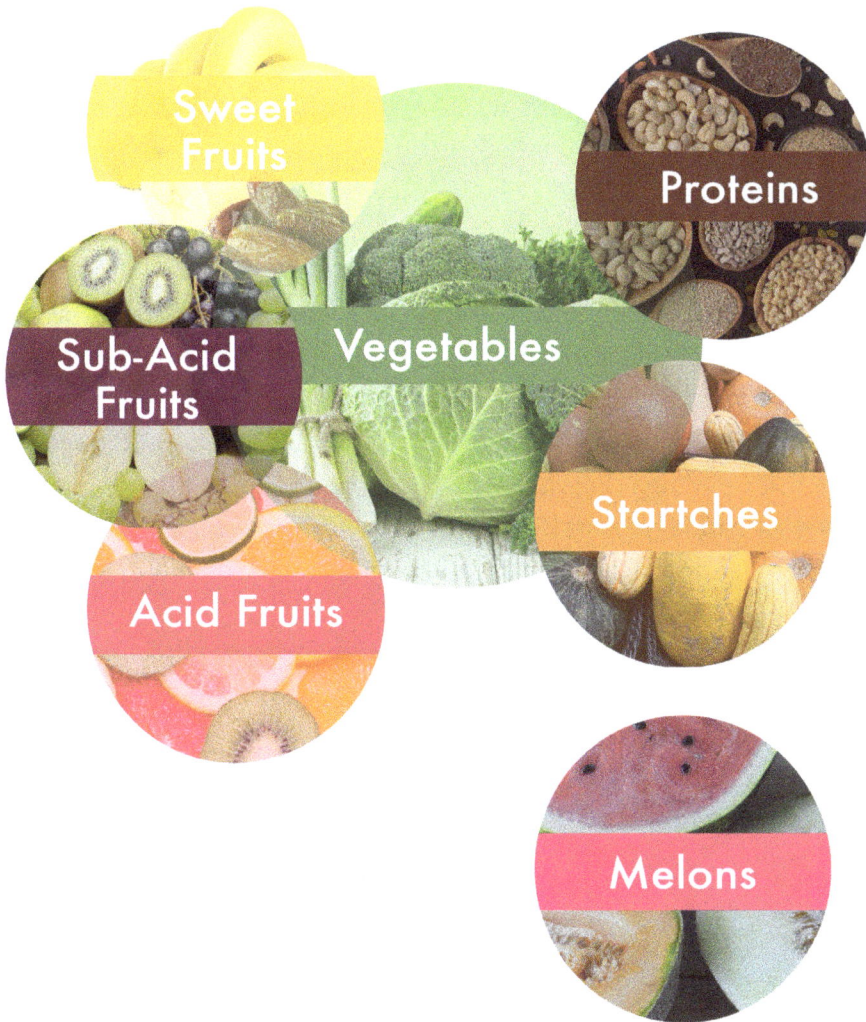

Learn to tap into what true satiety feels like to avoid overeating with conscious eating. Slow down, breathe, and give thanks before you eat. Remember that you are eating to live, not living to eat.

The Importance of Cleansing

Periodic cleansing is important for health and beauty. Even if you are eating cleaner than anybody else you know, you still need to cleanse your body. In the first few years of my cleansing journey, I was clearing out twenty-one years of toxins, chemicals, medications, negative emotions, and the remnants of processed foods. The internal channels of your body may become clogged and not function properly if you don't keep your internal body clean. Even if you are a healthy eater, periodic cleansing is like maintenance to keep your body in tip-top shape. It's like an oil change, keeping all systems clean and working properly.

The kidneys and the liver are in the body to remove toxins, but if those organs become toxic, this can lead to trouble. Over time, we are exposed to toxins through the environment, stress, beauty products, cleaning products, and food. Like taking out the trash or cleaning your house, your body is yours to live in. Look at the body from a functional standpoint. The systems are all connected: cardiovascular, endocrine, liver, colon, skin, and the nervous systems all work together, and if one is negatively affected, it can throw the whole system out of balance. If the villi within the colon are compromised, nutrients in food may not be absorbed and utilized to nourish and energize the body, mind, and spirit. The liver and colon affect many other functions in the body to a fascinating degree.

Cleansing allows the body to reset itself by removing the foods and beverages that might cause problems for individuals. There are different ways to cleanse. Some are gentler than others. It is up to you what you want to try. I recommend juice fasting, replacing unhealthy meals with smoothies, and whole food cleansing. Whole food cleanses are great for people who are not willing to juice fast. You would be eating clean whole foods for a period while leaving out offenders like coffee, alcohol, gluten, dairy, and processed sugar. It may sound difficult, but I assure you, the food can be prepared deliciously and the results are worth it! I offer a twenty-one day whole foods cleanse if you're interested!

The body's largest organ of elimination is the skin, and skin disorders are a problem for many people. How many times have you heard that acne is genetic? It is true that we are born with certain gene types that predispose us to certain conditions. This implies that you were born with something you cannot change and that you just have to accept the cards you have been dealt. This is true, we are born with DNA that we cannot change, but those genes are either turned on or off by lifestyle triggers. Genes are expressed depending on how a person lives, taking into consideration diet, lifestyle, and stress management. If you are genetically predisposed to acne or heart disease, you must be strategic about how you live and eat to ensure those genes are not expressed.

Acne is just a sign that something is wrong internally or off balance. It could be that your pores are clogged with the wrong skin care/makeup regimen, or you are reacting to a food intolerance. Acne is a huge problem not just for teenagers but for some adults as well. The causes of acne vary and are controversial. Getting to the root cause of a person's acne is different from person to person but essential to really curing it. How many times have you heard or read that diet does not affect acne? This is false. How could what you eat not affect your health? The skin is not exempt and is an outer reflection of what is going on internally and emotionally. The good, old phrase, "You are what you eat," is 100% valid. What you eat affects everything, though it is not the only factor that comes into play for great health and beauty.

Eating fruits and vegetables, nuts, seeds and sprouts is the BEST way to naturally look amazing. The vitamins, minerals, and nutrients in plants provide everything you need to look your best. Dairy products interfere with this ideal for many because those types of foods are clogging and mucus forming. In addition, dairy products have been linked to inflammation, which leads to skin conditions like acne and eczema. Many people attest to the fact that dairy products aggravate their skin breakouts, and by eliminating them, their skin conditions improved tremendously. This step is one of the most important steps necessary to enhance your glow.

Our appetite can be deceiving because what we want to eat isn't always what we need. A lot of times, we feel hunger when we are just thirsty, or we have some sort of emotional need that calls us to numb it with food. If you are craving unhealthy foods, perhaps you have been conditioned to eat that way. Instead, decode these cravings to give the body what it really needs, and sometimes that is love not pastries, space from toxic relationships not beer, or green juice and vegetables. A little quality dark chocolate helps, too! Learn to replace those unhealthy foods with healthy alternatives. Remember your mind is really what is in control of your body. Trust me, you will not miss the terrible feeling of regret, thinking, "Why did I eat that? Now I am suffering."

Probiotics are live microorganisms that live inside your intestines. The idea that depression causes a disturbance in gut health or vice versa is striking, and if gut health affects the skin, then addressing gut issues is addressing the root of many ailments. Stress, diet, antibiotics, yeast, parasites and more cause negative changes in the gut calling for restoration and rebalance. Gut health is associated with both anxiety and depression since any imbalance or inflammation in the gut can play a role in mental health. Probiotics could rebalance the gut and are essential to consume if you are experiencing depression, anxiety, inflammation or skin problems. In fact, probiotics had similar effects to antidepressants, reduces cortisol levels and improved psychological effects for participants in a study about the gut-brain axis.[10] Probiotic rich foods include yogurt, fermented vegetables, sauerkraut, and kimchi. Getting to the root cause of acne may take some time, so if you struggle with it, prepare to have patience in healing it. Probiotics help to eliminate inflammation (which plays a role in acne) as well as enhance nutrient absorption because they provide healthy bacteria to the gut.

---

10   Clapp, M., Aurora, N., Herrera, L., Bhatia, M., Wilen, E., & Wakefield, S. (2017). Gut microbiota's effect on mental health: The gut-brain axis. Clinics and Practice, 7(4), 987. http://doi.org/10.4081/cp.2017.987

CHAPTER 5
SUGAR:
THE NOT-SO-SWEET TRUTH

Are you ready for a sweet surrender? Sometimes the things in life we love the most are the very things we need to let go of to thrive, heal, and flourish. This idea of pruning excess and letting go allows us to practice self-control and blossom into the beauty that lays within each one of us. Saying "no" to processed sugar allows you to say "yes" to beauty and wellbeing. Let's face it. This is not something we want to hear because sugar tastes good and it stimulates the pleasure center in the brain, making it extremely addictive! Having it occasionally is okay for some people. For others, like myself, foregoing processed sugar is a way of life. I have done away with processed sugar and, I have to say, I don't feel like I'm missing out on anything. Fruit sugar is okay because fruit is extremely beneficial and life-giving in many ways. Additionally, fruit is recognized as food, contains water and fiber, and can be fully utilized by the body. For health and beauty purposes, we are concerned with processed forms of sugar and, surprisingly so, even more natural forms of sugar like honey and alcohol. Alcohol turns into sugar after it is consumed and creates a toxic load on the liver, which is why it's not good to have when trying to control inflammation.

You might be surprised to discover how much added sugar is in the foods people consume daily. Not only does processed sugar consumption lead to disease, but studies show that it is just as addictive as narcotics. Over a hundred peer reviewed articles showed that humans produce opioids – the chemically active ingredient in heroin, cocaine and other narcotics stemming from the digestion of excess sugars and fats.[11] As researchers examined the process by which the opioids are produced within the body, they notice addictive pattern behaviors. This binge behavior creates a "biochemically addictive process" with foods (processed sugar) that engage the brain in the same ways alcohol and addictive drugs do.[12] Sugar is addictive in similar ways to narcotics, and it is added unnecessarily to so many foods. Available evidence in humans shows that sugar and sweetness can induce biological rewards and cravings that are comparable in magnitude to those induced by addictive drugs such as

---

11   Cheren, M., Foushi, M., Helga Gudmundsdotter, E., Hillock, C., Lerner, M., Prager, M., Rice, M., Walsh, L., Werdell, P. *Physical Craving and Food Addiction,* Food Addiction Institute, 2009. .

12   Avena, N. M., Rada, P., & Hoebel, B. G. (2008). Evidence for sugar addiction: Behavioral and neurochemical effects of intermittent, excessive sugar intake. *Neuroscience and Biobehavioral Reviews,* 32(1), 20–39. http://doi.org/10.1016/j.neubiorev.2007.04.019

cocaine.[13] A can of soda alone has thirty-nine grams of sugar or more. Sugar is also added to foods like tomato sauce and yogurts unnecessarily. A reasonable sugar intake for a drink, protein powder, or snack is anything less than twelve grams.

Realizing the addictive properties of sugar shows just how powerful it is and why people are hooked! Sugar activates a reward sensation in the brain coupled with a temporary energy boost. This leads people, especially children, to seek it out in the same way they would other reward activities. The problem is that sugar is devoid of nutrition and leads to weight gain and tooth decay among other problems. While sugar may not exactly be in the same league as narcotics like cocaine and heroin, we should not dismiss the importance of sugar moderation, and we should be considering appropriate levels of consumption based on individual tolerance levels. When people come off sugar, they experience withdrawal effects like anger, moodiness, and even depression. Once that subsides, they are rewarded with stable moods, weight loss, and clear skin.

Nature did not intend for us to eat processed foods and the repercussions are tremendous. Childhood diabetes has been on the rise for years, and diabetes in general is a national epidemic in America. Even though sugar is not the actual cause of type 2 diabetes, it can certainly exacerbate it. People become addicted to the sweet taste sugar offers, but after a time of cutting it out, the palate changes and will begin to appreciate the taste of natural foods. You would be surprised at how insanely sweet some of the most popular coffee shop drinks taste after you get used to an unsweetened palate. Some of these drinks pack over fifty grams of sugar a pop! Sugar also leads to unstable blood sugar, mood swings, fatigue, and cravings.

What do we notice about highly processed foods that are low-fat or high-fat? They are loaded with sugar. Low-fat foods are notorious for having more sugar than high-fat foods since the removal of fat is replaced with the addition of sugar. Everyone has their own level of sugar tolerance, but let's face it, less to none is best for everyone! Your goal is to find out what your level of sugar tolerance is. Once you become aware of the symptoms of a sugar intolerance, you may find that yours is quite low. Many people look and feel much better by avoiding added sugar in foods. You will notice, once you get in the habit of reading labels on food items, that even "healthy" foods like yogurt, granola bars, and organic fruit snacks are loaded with added sugar. One serving of yogurt can contain up to twenty-two grams of sugar, which is higher than some servings of ice cream. Sugar also hides out in beverages like almond milk and rice milk. Always go for the unsweetened versions. Avoiding pack-

13 Ahmed, SH., Guillem, K., Vandaele, Y., *Sugar Addiction: pushing the drug-sugar analogy to the limit*, Curr Opin Clin Nutr Metab Care. 2013 July. 16(4):434-9. www.ncbi.nlm.nih.gov/pubmed/23719144

aged foods makes it easy to avoid added sugar in your diet.

Inflammation in the body is another concern associated with sugar consumption. Arthritis, cardiovascular disease, diabetes, acne, and memory loss are all contributed to by inflammation, therefore, sugar plays a key role here. Processed sugar is inflammatory, empty in nutritional value, contributes to obesity, diabetes, inflammation, and heart disease. Sugar exacerbates acne. When your body cannot process ingested sugar properly, it will affect the clarity of your skin. Have you ever thought that you had to avoid fruit or natural fruit juice to avoid carbohydrates or sugar? Abstaining from fruit and fruit juice for some time may be beneficial as well to help clear up any issues with candidiasis, hormonal imbalance, or to simply help your body rebalance its system. This includes avoiding natural forms of sugar like honey and maple syrup. If candidiasis or blood sugar issues are a problem, low glycemic fruits are good to have, such as berries, kiwi, and green apples.

The food industry doesn't make it easy for people who are avoiding sugar since it is present in a myriad of processed foods and drinks. Even foods appearing to be "healthy" can be high in organic cane sugar and other forms of sugar coined by names that people do not recognize as sugar. Do not be fooled. Just because the ingredient is listed as organic sugar doesn't mean it's all good. Processed sugar is sugar! Even healthier forms of sugar are still processed and need to be taken in moderation. Sugar no longer necessarily goes by its name as "sugar" on food labels. Therefore, whole food nutrition is the best way to navigate away from any forms of processed sugar because the sweet stuff is quite sneaky. Here some of the different names sugar goes by.

- Agave Nectar
- Barley Malt
- Beet Sugar
- Blackstrap Molasses
- Brown Rice Syrup
- Brown Sugar
- Buttered Sugar
- Cane Juice
- Cane Juice Crystals
- Caramel
- Carob Syrup
- Caster Sugar
- Coconut Sugar
- Confectioner's Sugar
- Corn Sweetener
- Corn Syrup
- Corn Syrup Solids
- Crystaline fructose
- Damerara Sugar
- Date Sugar
- Dextran
- Diastatic Malt
- Diatase
- Ethyl Maltol
- Evaporated Cane Juice
- Fructose

- Fruit Juice Concentrates
- Galactose
- Glucose
- Golden Sugar
- Golden Syrup
- High Fructose Corn Syrup
- Honey
- Invert Sugar
- Lactose
- Malt Syrup
- Maltodextrin
- Maltose
- Maple Syrup
- Molasses Syrup
- Muscovado Sugar
- Oat Syrup
- Organic Raw Sugar
- Panela
- Panocha
- Rice Bran Syrup
- Rice Syrup
- Sorghum Syrup
- Sucrose
- Sugar
- Syrup
- Tapioca Syrup
- Treacle
- Turbinado Sugar
- Yellow Sugar

Sugar contributes to other health issues like type 2 diabetes (which can be reversed and controlled by controlling sugar intake). Forget about using artificial sweeteners like Splenda, aspartame, acesulfame-K, saccharin, and sucralose. They are hundreds of times sweeter than sugar, and studies suggest that they may be linked to type 2 diabetes.[14] Artificial sweeteners trick your brain into thinking it's getting sugar but without the calories. The problem with this trickery is it causes people to crave more sweet foods and drinks, which adds up to extra calories in the end and possibly weight gain. Artificial sweeteners may impair the body's response to glucose, therefore, the body is not controlling blood sugar properly. This sounds a lot like what happens with diabetes.

Since artificial sweeteners are linked to obesity and obesity is linked to diabetes, we can see a connection. Another study showed that the people who drank artificially sweetened drinks had a 47% higher increase in BMI than those who did not.[15] In recipes, coconut nectar and coconut sugar are great alternatives to processed sugars. Coconut sugar is low glycemic and has minerals. I love using dates or adding liquid stevia to recipes when I want something sweet. Dates are a fruit and a whole food, so they are completely unprocessed, sweet, delicious, and contain fiber. Stevia comes from a plant and is not an artificial chemical sweetener. It's best to avoid artificial, chemical sweeteners completely. You can soak dates in some filtered water for a few hours which makes them soft

14   Carbohydrate metabolism and diabetes: Guy Fagherazzi, Alice Vilier, Daniela Saes Sartorelli, Martin Lajous, Beverley Balkau, and Françoise Clavel-Chapelon

15   Harvard T.H. Chan (2018). School of Public Health. Artificial Sweeteners. Retrieved from www.hsph.harvard.edu/nutritionsource/healthy-drinks/artificial-sweeteners

and easy to blend. Adding dates to smoothies and recipes is a great way to add sweetness without adding processed sugar. Not only are they low glycemic (thirty-five on the scale), but they are vegan and nutritious as well, providing vitamin C and B vitamins. Agave and maple syrup are popular vegan sweeteners but are more heavily processed.

Spikes in blood sugar lead to blood sugar imbalances. This affects a person's mood and mental state. Depression can occur after the blood sugar rises and then drops after eating white, refined carbohydrates and sugars. Sugar is that powerful, and rats in studies showed signs of sugar withdrawal such as stress, nervousness, and anxiety just as people addicted to drugs like nicotine and morphine would.[16] Research also shows that, when given the option, rats choose sugar over cocaine.[17]

Increased sugar consumption has doubled since 1980 and has contributed to a worldwide epidemic of obesity. The American Psychological Association reports the United States spends $71 billion dollars on treating depressive disorders, right under $101 billion for diabetes.[18] Imagine what the nation could do with that money if people were treating this atrocity with lifestyle changes, diet, exercise, meditation, and alternative methods when appropriate and possible. The side effects of many of the medications given to people with depression are scary. I once heard a famous doctor say depression is not a Prozac deficiency, and a headache is not an aspirin deficiency. Asking oneself what is causing this depression or headache helps to solve the problem, not mask it. Choose lifestyle changes when possible, not pills.

When setting out to avoid sugar, remember that fruit does not count as harmful sugar! Fruit is a whole food and consists of water, nutrients and fiber, which slow down the release of sugar into the bloodstream. Our bodies need carbohydrates to function and our brains thrive off them. Carbohydrates are broken down into sugar and used for energy. Not all carbs are created equal, however, and depriving your body of them is not a good idea. Fruit is the perfect carbohydrate fuel.

Refined or simple carbohydrates come from processed sugars found in foods like cookies, candies, and commercial yogurts and pasta sauce. They enter the bloodstream very quickly because they have already been broken down. Complex carbohydrates come from fruit, starchy vegetables, and grains such as oatmeal and brown rice. They are broken down and released slowly into the blood-

16   Princeton University. "Sugar Can Be Addictive: Animal Studies Show Sugar Dependence." Science Daily. ScienceDaily, 11 December 2008.
17   Lenoir M. Serre F, Cantin L, Ahmed SH (2007) Intense Sweetness Surpasses Cocaine Reward. PLoS ONE 2(8):e698.doi:10.1371/journal.pone.0000698
18   Winerman, L. (2017). The American Psychological Association. By the numbers: The cost of treatment. Retrieved from http://www.apa.org/monitor/2017/03/numbers.aspx

stream to provide stable energy. There are small amounts of carbohydrates in most green vegetables, which is why they may be eaten in abundance and help stabilize blood sugar levels. The glycemic index gives a value of sugar amounts in food and is used to help people gauge the amount of sugar in the foods they eat. The glycemic load is another number which gives the value of how the food will impact a person's blood sugar levels after eating it. You will see that the glycemic load of fruit is actually low. Foods with a low glycemic load have a number of 10 or lower, medium is 11-19, and foods scoring 20 or more are considered high. Watermelon is relatively high on the glycemic index with a rating of 80, however, it is low in carbohydrates, so its glycemic load is only around 5-7. Here is a chart comparing the glycemic index to the glycemic load in foods.

Glycemic Load vs. Glycemic Index[19]

Vegetables	Glycemic Index	Glycemic Load
Potato	104	97
Carrot	39	2
Yellow Corn	48	14
Sweet Potato	70	22
Yam	54	20
Tomato	38	1.5
Green Peas	54	20
Parsnips	52	4
Broccoli	0	0
Cabbage	0	0
Celery	0	0
Cauliflower	0	0
Green Beans	0	0
Mushrooms	0	0
Spinach	0	0
Kale	0	0

19   Atkinson, Foster-Powell, & Brand-Miller, International tables of glycemic index and glycemic load values: 2008, Diabetes Care, Vol. 31, number 12, pgs. 2281-2283.

Fruit	Glycemic Index	Glycemic Load
Watermelon	72	7.2
Pineapple	66	11.9
Cantaloupe	65	7.8
Papaya	60	6.6
Raisins	64	20.5
Banana	48	11
Mango	51	12.8
Orange	48	7.2
Pears	38	4
Grapes	43	6.5
Strawberries	40	3.6
Blueberries	40	5
Dates	42	18
Apples	36	5
Dried Apricot	32	23
Apricot	31	3
Prunes	29	10
Peach	28	2.2
Grapefruit	25	2.8
Plum	22	1.7
Cherries	22	3.7
Nuts	**Glycemic Index**	**Glycemic Load**
Cashews	22	0
Most Nut Varieties	0	0

Many people are afraid of eating carbs and severely restrict them in an effort to lose weight. But is that truly healthy or sustainable long-term? Balance is sustainable, healthy, and unrestrictive. Don't be afraid to eat fruits or complex carbohydrates as a part of a healthy lifestyle! They will not make you fat and you will feel happier and more energetic. Say *no* to highly refined carbohydrates like white flour and sugar or consume them in moderation. Once you have been off refined sugars for a while, you will feel a difference after eating them again that may cause you to give them up completely. You have nothing to lose and everything to gain.

CHAPTER 6
COFFEE: FRIEND OR FOE?

Millions of people think they cannot live without coffee nor do they want to as it is one of the most popular beverages worldwide. The aroma of this delicious drink, brewed to perfection, entertains our senses, bringing a sense of happiness to the psyche. There is no debate that coffee tastes and smells amazing. I will, hands down, admit that I love hemp milk lattes. I wish they loved me back. The jolt of energy, mental alertness, and elevated feelings we get from drinking coffee brings us to brew it daily or visit our favorite coffee shops. Among Americans, nearly 50% (150 million people) drink around three cups of coffee a day.[20] Despite its popularity, there are health issues associated with caffeine consumption, like hormonal imbalance, acne, anxiety, and adrenal fatigue. For all the avid coffee lovers out there, you've got ninety-nine problems, and you don't want coffee to be one!

There are studies proving many of the benefits coffee has to offer. Who doesn't want more "energy," an elevated mood, increased mental focus, and the simple pleasure in having a cup? While there are pros associated with drinking coffee and caffeine, there are also some concerns worth considering, like increased cortisol levels, high blood pressure, drops in blood sugar levels, weight gain, consistent food cravings, breakouts, upset stomach, acid reflux, anxiety, and more. These are some of the side effects associated with consumption of this boisterous beverage. When I am on the go and my schedule is packed, I notice that having caffeine upsets my stomach and I feel a crash followed by anxiety, sometimes with dizziness, a few hours after drinking it. It feels as if my blood sugar drops significantly. When I don't drink coffee, these things almost never occur. After a few years of unravelling this beast, I noticed that daily coffee consumption caused my hormones to become imbalanced and I would get breakouts along my chin and jawline. After a week or more without it, my skin clears and my anxiety fades away. The connection was made and now I choose more sleep and relaxation over a coffee crutch whenever possible.

The key is to remember that everyone is different in terms of caffeine sensitivity. We also

---

20   Coffee consumption statistics. (2017) Retrieved from http://www.e-importz.com/coffee-statistics.php

all experience different environmental stressors and have different genetic makeups. These things can alter our caffeine sensitivity as well. Some people reap the benefits of coffee with little-to-no problems while others cannot. It's highly beneficial to closely examine any symptoms you are having that could be associated with coffee and caffeine consumption. If you don't want to give it up, then find an amount you can tolerate.

Coffee is acidic and, at one time, the acid reflux I was experiencing felt like I was being strangled at the neck. I had to remove coffee and other acidic foods from my diet for six weeks to be relieved of acid reflux. Once I did that, the reflux subsided and I was relieved. Now I can enjoy an occasional cup of organic coffee here and there without suffering. Personally, I found that even one latte a day consistently disrupts my digestion, blood sugar stability, and hormonal health. I'm better off having it once in a blue moon or once a week and sticking to tea instead.

Caffeine is a legal drug of choice and many are addicted. When you come off coffee, you will feel the withdrawal symptoms, for sure! However, you might be surprised at how much better you look and feel when coming off this drug. Consider whether caffeine is your friend or your foe. Keep in mind your tolerance level may depend on the day, your health, and/or current stress levels. Coffee raises cortisol levels. Cortisol is known as the stress hormone, and high levels of cortisol in the body can lead to health atrocities such as increased weight gain (especially around the midsection), high blood pressure, lower cognitive functioning, high cholesterol, and lower immune function. There are times in life when stress is high, and the absence of coffee and caffeine is essential to keep cortisol levels and inflammation down.

Caffeine also causes problems for maintaining blood sugar stability, which increases insulin levels and contributes to stress and anxiety. This may cause you to feel shaky, dizzy, spacy, or even anxious after drinking it. Caffeinated coffee has been shown to create insulin resistance in healthy, obese, and type 2 diabetic people.[21] More insulin in the blood makes you feel less than your best, and I personally have experienced insulin sensitivity with caffeinated coffee consumption. I notice when I have green or black tea instead of coffee, I do not feel anxious and experience a calmer mind. Forgoing the cup of joe increases beauty, energy levels, decreases anxiety, and stabilizes blood sugar. Feeling more grounded and peaceful helps me to react to stressors in a more positive way and this makes life run more smoothly. When stress hormones are not running rampant in the system, caffeine will not exacerbate inflammation. This could be due to having more time to relax, sleep, and eat

21   Moisey LL, Kacker S, Bickerton AC, Robinson LE, Graham TE. (2008), "Caffeinated coffee consumption impairs blood glucose homeostasis in response to high and low glycemic index meals in healthy men." American Journal of Clinical Nutrition. 87 (5):1254-1261.

properly. Think of having a latte as a treat rather than a daily necessity.

People especially love coffee or caffeine before a workout or study session for mental or physical stamina. Adding coconut oil to your coffee helps avoid a crash since the fat slows down the caffeine release in the bloodstream. I encourage you to abstain from coffee for thirty days so you can decide if coffee is for or against you. I also find that I sleep better at night when I don't drink caffeine, and sleep is not something to skimp on or take lightly.

All too often, we think we can get by on far too little. Having coffee after the noon hours or into the evening can interfere with sleep patterns and lead to insomnia, which perpetuates the cycle of "needing" coffee in the morning to wake up. Interrupted sleep patterns lead to a cycle of sleep deprivation thus feeding the addiction. If you are going to have a cup, morning is the best time. You may experience increased hunger in efforts to stabilize blood sugar, or feel shaky or irritable hours after consumption. The message here is not "all or nothing," and you certainly do not have to give up coffee and caffeine forever. At times, it is a good idea to stay away from it to achieve cleansing, to balance your hormones, rest the adrenal glands, or clear up issues with anxiety and skin problems. You may find that giving it up altogether is best for your health and beauty.

Recently, a client shared with me that her coworkers noticed her energy levels skyrocketing. When they asked her what she was doing, she said she gave up coffee! This is not what you might expect to hear. She works twelve-hour days as an oncology nurse and is now working out afterwards and walking her dogs. She also shared with me that her blood sugar has stabilized, and she lost four pounds in one week by switching to more plant-based smoothies and meals. She abstained from coffee and alcohol—two things she was previously addicted to. Switching to green tea is a great alternative for coffee and offers high levels of beauty preserving antioxidants. Other coffee alternatives include Dandy Blend, black tea, oolong tea, Pero, white tea, and yerba mate.

We were created to live healthfully and with enough energy to live our lives without being dependent on medications and addictive substances like coffee. Caffeine is present in different products like energy drinks, chocolate, soda, and coffee. Caffeine is consumed in different ways that stimulates a kind of artificial energy in our bodies that can lead to heart palpitations. The energy we feel from caffeine is given to us like borrowed money on credit. Our bodies become hyper-stimulated and we use that false energy to run ourselves into the ground. We must pay for it eventually, and then some. Rest, relaxation, and sleep is necessary for our body to naturally restore itself. If that's not happening, we pay the price with more fatigue, mood swings, food cravings, and less overall beauty.

Let's talk about caffeine and the adrenal glands. The adrenal glands are two small organs that sit above the kidneys. They release the hormones cortisol and adrenaline, which prepare one for a fight or flight situation. Prolonged caffeine consumption and a lack of sleep can wear out these glands and prevent them from functioning properly. This is called adrenal fatigue (and most commonly occurs in women). There are ways to combat the fatigue and support the body rather than hinder it. Supplements such as vitamin C, D-ribose, vitamin B-5, magnesium, and ashwagandha help restore energy levels. Ashwagandha is an adaptogen that is good for balancing hormones by reducing stress levels and increasing physical performance in users. This reduces anxiety and cortisol levels, which helps with stress related depression as well. D-ribose has been found through research to effectively reduce symptoms of chronic fatigue syndrome associated with adrenal fatigue.[22]

Aside from the health benefits of having or not having coffee, let us not forget about the beauty benefits. By eliminating caffeine for cleansing or lifestyle purposes, you may notice that you are calmer, your skin clears up, your moods even out, you have less food cravings, and your face appears refreshed and younger looking. Replace your morning coffee with a green juice and you will notice how you look and feel rejuvenated and refreshed. Having better sleep boosts beauty dramatically. It's call "beauty sleep" for a reason. When insulin and cortisol are not wreaking havoc in the body, you feel calmer and happier. Guess what? Having a calm and happy state of mind will help you look better too. Feeling tired, cranky, and frazzled never looks good on anyone. For whatever reason, when I have caffeine daily, even organic coffee, my skin breaks out. Clear, healthy skin is a sign of beauty and health. This is yet another example of how forgoing the joe can increase beauty.

---

22   Teitelbaum JE1, Johnson C, St Cyr J. The Use of D-ribose in Chronic Fatigue Syndrome and Fibromyalgia: a pilot study. J Altern Complement Med. 2006 Nov;12(9):857-62.

CHAPTER 7
NOT YOUR MOTHER'S MILK

Milk does the body good. Says who? Milk is a sacred liquid created by a mother to feed and nourish her baby. Think about the process of breastfeeding, as it is one that is intimate and bonding in nature between a mother and child. This is how nature designed milk to be used, for mother and offspring of similar species. The human species is the only species that continues consuming milk after the weaning stages of life. People began consuming milk thousands of years ago in Northern and Eastern regions of Europe after the domestication of animals began. Romans used sheep and goat milk to make cheese and yogurt. Why are humans are still drinking milk long after the Industrial Revolution? If you lived in rural Russia hundreds of years ago and a cow lived in your backyard, it would make sense to milk the cow and use what was readily available for survival. Humanity has evolved and it is no longer necessary to use animals to produce products we are accustomed to, like milk for example.

People could stop consuming dairy products for health, ethical, and beauty reasons. Despite this, consuming dairy products has been the norm and continues out of tradition, unawareness, and convenience. Because milk, cheese, ice cream, and pizza have always been popular American foods, people continue eating these cultural favorites without thinking anything of it. People are still consuming a beverage that was created to rear a calf, meant to grow into a 1500-pound animal. The American government promotes dairy products and enlists educational programs in schools to educate children about the health benefits of dairy. Milk is served in schools to children nationwide and it is consumed by Americans daily in gallons. Why aren't school children being taught the truth, which is that plants provide all the nutrition you will ever need to build strong bones and be healthy? America seems convinced that dairy products are necessary to build strong bones and provide ample nutrition due to successful dairy lobbying. Milk could provide nutrition; however, the dairy industry sold $9.4 billion dollars' worth of milk in 2014, and made about 21 billion worth of revenue. This leads one to believe that milk and dairy products are massed produced for profit.

The dairy industry contributes to the economy, but at the expense of what? What if instead the dairy lobbying funds were redirected towards organic farmers and we switched gears to convince children among the masses that plants could meet their dietary needs? Could America be a healthier nation, contributing to less animal cruelty? If milk were necessary for the good health of humans, why is are so many people lactose intolerant? Overall, about 75 percent of the world's population, including 25 percent of those in the U.S., lose their lactase enzymes after weaning.[23]

Nutritionists, doctors, and the National Dairy Council encourage people to include dairy products in their diet. On the other hand, numerous nutritionists, health experts, and doctors like T. Colin Campbell, Neal Barnard, Dean Ornish, Joel Fuhrman, and Gabriel Cousens disagree. Despite milk's nutritional profile, by choosing not to drink milk, you are not missing out on nutrients like vitamin D, protein, potassium, and calcium. It's not as if those nutrients are not available elsewhere. In fact, many milk alternatives are fortified with calcium. For example, Califia Farms almond milk has 50% more calcium than dairy milk, and the unsweetened variety only has forty calories per serving. Vitamin D is often fortified in foods like cereals, orange juice, and plant-based milks. Bananas are loaded with potassium, and protein can be found in numerous plants such as vegetables, nuts, seeds, and legumes.

T.Colin Campbell, in his book, *The China Study,* references years' worth of studies showing a correlation between dairy products and disease. Dairy products are thought to be linked to a myriad of health problems such as acne, food allergies, cancer, heart disease, diabetes, inflammation, and contaminant exposure (hormones, drugs, and pesticides), and asthma. A lot of well-meaning nutritionists teach that milk is an excellent beverage, providing essential nutrients such as vitamin D, protein, and calcium. Without vitamin D, only a small amount of calcium can be absorbed. A misconception is that milk is necessary to provide dietary vitamin D, but this is not true. A few foods contain this vitamin naturally. The body produces its own vitamin D with fifteen minutes of direct sunlight, and supplements are always available. Lamps for light therapy are also an option for people who do not live in sunny climates. This is useful because vitamin D deficiency is associated with depression, and light therapy and sunshine are effective remedies.

Lactose intolerance is one of the reasons why Americans are shifting away from dairy product consumption. Signs of dairy and lactose intolerance include gas, bloating, intestinal cramping, and diarrhea. Products like pills and lactose-free milk are on the market to help to relieve and/or avoid these symptoms. If you are lactose intolerant, why take pills? It is a better idea to forgo the dairy products altogether and not have to think about one more thing like purchasing a pill, needing to have it on hand when you want to eat something containing dairy, and spending extra money on the pill.

23 Hertzler, S.R, Huynh BCL, Savaiano DA. How much lactose is low lactose? *J Am Dietetic Asso.* 1996;96:243-246.

A2 milk was developed as an alternative for people who have a difficult time digesting milk. The a2 protein present in milk with the absence of the a1 protein does not seem to cause problems for people with lactose intolerance. It is pasteurized and free of growth hormones, coming from cows that only produce the a2 protein. A1 protein came about as the result of a genetic mutation in domestic cows thousands of years ago, and it spread throughout Europe and the United States. Most cows carry both the a1 and a2 proteins, however, scientists believe that the a1 protein is the culprit for causing lactose intolerance and/or gassy, queasy, bloated feelings felt in people without lactose intolerance. This is a debatable topic, but the premise is that a2 milk more closely resembles the milk that was consumed centuries ago.[24] Even a2 milk, like all milk, contains casein, which is another reason why dairy is problematic. Casein is a milk protein in dairy products, and cheese is especially high in it. Dr. Neal Barnard mentions in his book *The Cheese Trap* that cheese is helping make people overweight and sick, and it triggers inflammation. Dr. Bernard also states that giving up cheese could bring relief to asthma symptoms.[25] Casein digests slowly, which causes digestive problems. It also has addictive properties due to morphine-like substances released into the bloodstream. People become addicted to dairy products like cheese and ice cream, just as they do sugar and meat.[26] Just like with any addictive substance, when abstaining from it, withdrawal symptoms could arise like mood swings.

Dr. T. Colin Campbell deems casein as promoting cancer. Though cancer begins with genetics, casein and animal proteins were found to turn on cancer growth, while plant proteins did not.[27] There are also studies stacked up against dairy products linking them to cancer,[28] diabetes,[29] acne,[30] bone fractures,[31] ear infections, constipation, multiple sclerosis, prostate cancer, and higher ovarian cancer risk.[32] Clearly there is nutritional value in milk, however if your body does not tolerate it and you experience any of the ailments associated with it, there is no sense in drinking it. Milk doesn't reduce fractures, and countries with the lowest consumption of dairy have the lowest rates of osteoporosis.

24   Could a2 Milk Solve Lactose Intolerance Symptoms for Some? NBC News, Better Diet and Fitness, April 2015, http://www.nbcnews.com/better/diet-fitness/can-new-milk-brand-buoy-dairy-industry-n339586

25   King, Barbara J. (2017) National Public Radio. Doctor's Book Presents the Case Against 'Dairy Crack'. Retrieved from https://npr.org/sections/13.7/2017/02/23/516779481/doctors-book-presents

26   Barnard, Neal D., MD. (2012) Brain Hijackers: The 4 Most Addictive Foods. Retrieved from https://www.doctoroz.com/article/brain-hijackers-4-most-addictive-foods

27   Carney, Linda MD. (2014) Animal Protein "Turns On" Cancer Genes. Retrieved from https://www.drcarney.com/blog/entry/animal-protein-turns-on-cancer-genes

28   Youngman LD, Campbell TC. Inhibition of aflatoxin B1-induced gamma-glutamyltranspeptidase positive (GGT+) hepatic preneoplastic foci and tumors by low protein diets: evidence that altered GGT+ foci indicate neoplastic potential. Carcinogenesis 1992;13:1607-13.

29   Youngman LD, Campbell TC. Inhibition of aflatoxin B1-induced gamma-glutamyltranspeptidase positive (GGT+) hepatic preneoplastic foci and tumors by low protein diets: evidence that altered GGT+ foci indicate neoplastic potential. Carcinogenesis 1992;13:1607-13.

30   Spencer EH, Ferdowsian HR, Barnard ND. Diet and acne: a review of the evidence. Int J Dermatol 2009;48:339-47.

31   Michaelsson K, Wolk A, Langenskiold S, et al. Milk intake and risk of mortality and fractures in women and men: cohort studies. Bmj 2014;349:g6015.

32   http://nutritionstudies.org/12-frightening-facts-milk/

These other factors could be regional differences in overall diet and lifestyle such as increased exposure to daily sunlight, and exercise. Countries like India, Japan, and Peru intake as little as 300 mg per day of calcium (less than a third of the US recommendation for adults) and those countries have a low occurrence of bone fractures.[33]

> **Accumulating evidence shows that consuming milk or dairy products may contribute to the risk of prostate and ovarian cancers, autoimmune diseases, and some childhood ailments. Because milk is not necessary for humans after weaning and the nutrients it contains are readily available in foods without animal protein, saturated fat, and cholesterol, vegetarians may have healthier outcomes for chronic disease if they limit or avoid milk and other dairy products. Bones are better served by attending to calcium balance and focusing efforts on increasing fruit and vegetable intakes, limiting animal protein, exercising regularly, getting adequate sunshine or supplemental vitamin D, and getting approximately 500 mg Ca/d from plant sources. Therefore, dairy products should not be recommended in a healthy vegetarian diet.[34]**

Contrary to the U.S. daily recommendations for calcium intake, adequate amounts have not actually been established. According to Harvard's School of Public Health, studies suggest that a high intake of calcium does not decrease the risk of osteoporosis.[35] In addition, another study found that calcium intake did not predict hip fracture risk even with calcium supplementation.[36] You can clearly see the benefits of discarding dairy from your diet, however, the buck doesn't stop there.

There are more reasons to cut out dairy products. Dr. Mark Hyman proclaims that milk products are bad for your health, and his writings led me to discover that Harvard scientists found no data supporting the claim that dairy leads to better bones, weight loss, or improved health. In the study, serious risks associated with dairy products were again increased cancer and fracture risk, weight gain, irritable bowel syndrome, allergies, gas, bloating, eczema, acne, and chronic constipation.[37]

---

33   Harvard T.H. Chan, School of Public Health, (2018) Calcium: What's Best for Your Bones and Health? Retrieved from https://www.hsph.harvard.edu/nutritionsource/what-should-you-eat/calcium-and-milk/calcium-full-story/

34   Lanou AJ. Should dairy be recommended as part of a healthy vegetarian diet? *Am J Clin Nutr.* 2009;89:1638S-1642S. https://www.hsph.harvard.edu/nutritionsource/calcium-full-story/

35   https://www.hsph.harvard.edu/nutritionsource/calcium-full-story/

36   Feskanich D, Willett WC, Stampfer MJ, Colditz GA. Milk, dietary calcium, and bone fractures in women: a 12-year prospective study. Am J Public Health. 1997; 87:992–97.

37   Ludwig DS, Willet WC. (2013) JAMA Pediatrician. Three Daily Servings of Reduced-Fat Milk an Evidence Based Recommendation? 167(9):788-789.doi:10.1001/jamapediatrics.2013.2408

I had always suffered from allergies throughout my life, but they became less severe as I gave up animal products and gluten. You will notice a stronger immune system with less coughs, colds, sneezes, and flus. If you cut out sugar, dairy, meat, and gluten, you just may find yourself well 90% of the time. In my experience, I do not get sick often, and if I feel something coming on, I can rest, drink some fresh juice and shots made of citrus, turmeric and ginger, and feel better in a day or two. After a year of eating raw-vegan, I have not suffered any flus, major colds or sicknesses, which is unlike previous years of eating cooked vegan foods.

Medications and hormones have been found in milk, casein, and conventional meat. In 2015, the FDA conducted studies to test the milk being produced by dairy farmers. Findings shed light on the fact that numerous medications were found in samples of milk, which has been the case since 1918 when milk was originally being tested for illegal drugs. Confirmed drug residues were identified in milk. The drugs that were found as confirmed residues in this milk survey have also been reported by FSIS (Food Safety Inspection Service) as tissue residues found in dairy cows.

None of the confirmed drug residues identified in this milk survey are currently required to be routinely tested for under the Pasteurized Milk Ordinance for Grade "A" milk and milk products. None of the drugs found in the targeted or non-targeted groups are approved by FDA to be administered to lactating dairy cows. This means that FDA has not evaluated the use of these drugs in lactating dairy cattle, including whether milk from treated cows is safe for human consumption.[38]

These are things to consider when making decisions about what foods to consume. It's much easier to believe advertising like, "Milk does the body good," with pictures of famous athletes and think it means that milk is something beneficial for your health. Health risks of milk and dairy products are not advertised, and if more people became educated and enlightened about these risks, supported by the media, more medical doctors and science, they would think differently about that slice of pizza or glass of milk.

Aside from the majority of people who are lactose intolerant, what about the folks who can have dairy products without any problems? Your ancestry may affect your ability to digest milk and dairy products. Many people in Eastern and Northern Europe have acquired a lactose tolerance, whereby they now have the genetic makeup necessary to tolerate milk. Research conducted by Professor Mark Thomas with UCL (University College London) Genetics, Evolution and Environment

---

38   Center for Veterinary Medicine. FDA Department of Health and Human Services. (2015) Milk and Drug Residue Sampling Survey. Retrieved from https://www.fda.gov/downloads/AnimalVeterinary/GuidanceComplianceEnforcement/ComplianceEnforcement/UCM435759.pdf

states that "most adults worldwide do not produce the enzyme lactase and so are unable to digest the milk sugar lactose. However, most Europeans continue to produce lactase throughout their life, a characteristic known as lactase persistence." This occurred as a genetic mutation that allowed people greater survival since dairy consumption began after the domestication of animals.[39] The concept of lactose persistence suggests there was a genetic change in the ability for Europeans to drink milk without getting sick. Milk used to make some of the first humans who began to consume it sick and they evolved genetically over thousands of years to tolerate it. This could explain why some people are fine with milk products and some are not.

Have you noticed how widespread and popular many plant-based milks have become lately? Though the masses still consume dairy, its consumption is on the decline in America. Due to this decline, many companies have created numerous delicious alternatives to dairy products that effortlessly take their place for baking, cooking, smoothies, coffee creamer, and butters. People are making a change. With alternative milk choices like almond, coconut, cashew, hemp, rice, and hazelnut milk, it really is quite easy to switch to an alternative to milk. In addition, many delicious dairy-free ice creams, bars, cheeses, "cheese" cakes, and other desserts are on the market, and they taste great!

Choosing dairy alternatives contributes to whole body thriving. It is worth your time to see for yourself how dairy affects your health and beauty. If you want clearer skin and better digestion, cut out dairy for one month and then reintroduce it. Notice any differences within a week and note how you feel. If excess weight is an issue for you, then cutting out dairy could help you lose the extra pounds or inches. By eating raw plant foods close to nature, you are setting yourself up for effortless health, energy, and beauty. Yes, there are low-fat and nonfat varieties of dairy products available, but this does not ease the strain on the body and the environment, nor does it do anything to stop the cruelty taking place to produce the dairy.

The dairy industry has deleterious effects on the environment and is cruel in nature. To keep cows continuously producing milk in unnatural amounts, farmers participate in the abuse and constant artificial insemination of cows. This practice perpetuates stealing baby cows from mothers at birth, continual forced pregnancy, infections, swollen udders, and pus existence in dairy products. Because cow udders are over producing milk, they become swollen and infected, and this creates the necessity for antibiotic use. Even though milk sold in stores is pasteurized, it still contains remnants of pus and that is what you are drinking if you choose to partake.[40] Although dairy farmers are viewing

39   Milk Drinking Started in Central Europe, Press Release, University College London, August 2009, https://www.ucl.ac.uk/news/news-articles/0908/09082801
40   M. Greger, M.D., "How Much Pus is There in Milk?", nutritionfacts.org/2011/09/08/how-much-pus-is-there-in-milk, September 2011.

animals merely as products, cows have feelings, and separating a baby cow from its mother at birth creates stress and sadness for the mother and baby.

Other cruel practices take place because of the dairy industry. Sadly, 21,000,000 calves are slaughtered for cheap veal and beef production in conjunction with the mass production of milk.[41] Calves are restricted to confinement and live in horrible conditions, bound by the neck in bare stalls, unable to move around and live out a natural life. A cow's lifespan is usually around twenty-five years, but after being used for up to four years, a cow's tired and abused body is slaughtered, and ends up as a meal on somebody's plate. Not only is this an issue of health, but also an issue of ethics. Ask yourself if you really want to support an industry of such practices. You won't miss a thing once you experience all that the plant-based food industry has to offer.

Instead of dairy ice cream, you can make banana "nice" cream (my personal favorite) from the recipe in this book. Companies like Almond Hill and Daiya make delicious yogurts, cheeses, frozen desserts, and pizzas that are not soy based for people transitioning to a plant-based diet. Countless people can lose weight, reverse heart disease, lower bad cholesterol, lower the risks of strokes, lower blood pressure, and decrease the risks of type 2 diabetes by following a vegan diet.

Giving up dairy was one of the final decisions I made in my transition to the vegan lifestyle and is one of the best decisions I've ever made! You may find this true for yourself as well. It is wise to examine the role that dairy products play in your health and beauty lifestyle. The questions to ask yourself are, "Does dairy serve me? And do I really need it in my life?" I would like you to seriously ponder these questions and think for yourself about what you are going to support when you spend your dollars in restaurants and grocery stores. It goes so much deeper than a milkshake or whole milk latte. It's about the pain, suffering, abuse, and ethics involved with producing dairy products. Animal products are not necessary to consume for good health, and many doctors live the vegan life-style. Among them are Dean Ornish, Micheal Greger, Neal Bernard, John A. McDougall, Joel Fuhrman, Micheal Klaper, and Gabriel Cousins.

Calcium is an important nutrient people are concerned about when considering the vegan diet. As children, we were taught to drink milk to build strong bones because of the calcium content in dairy foods. While dairy products do contain protein and calcium, studies do not support that dairy product consumption reduces the risk of osteoporosis or bone fractures. Contrary to the belief that

---

41   "Calf Slaughter by Country in 1,000 Head," Index Mundi: Animal Numbers. Accessed 7/21/2014 from: http://www.indexmundi.com/agriculture/?commodity=cattle&graph=calf-slaughter

milk builds strong bones, clinical studies show no protective effect of increased milk consumption on fracture risk.[42] The National Academy of Sciences recommends 1000 mg/day for ages 19-50 and 1,200 mg for those 50 and older.

The amount of calcium we need is debatable, but the fact that we need it is not. You can increase bone density and decrease the risk of osteoporosis with exercise, and these benefits have been observed in studies of both children and adults.[43] Other ways to increase bone health include getting vitamins A, K, and D (from sunlight, fortified foods, or supplements), eating leafy greens, and weight bearing/strengthening exercise.

Here is a chart listing plant-based sources of calcium based on a 3.5 ounce portion size:

Plant Based Calcium Sources

Sesame Seeds	1160 mg
Amaranth	267 mg
Collard Greens	250 mg
Kale	249 mg
Almonds	234 mg
Parsley	203 mg
Dandelion Greens	187 mg
Mustard Greens	183 mg
Watercress	151 mg
Chickpeas	150 mg
Beans	135 mg
Pistachio Nuts	131 mg
Figs	126 mg
Sunflower Seeds	120 mg
Buckwheat	114 mg
Beet Greens	99 mg

42   Feskanich D, Willett WC, Colditz GA. Calcium, vitamin D, milk consumption, and hip fractures: a prospective study among postmenopausal women. Am J Clin Nutr. 2003;77:504–511. http://www.pcrm.org/sites/default/files/pdfs/health/Nutrition-Fact-Sheets/Dairy-Fact-Sheet.pdf
43   Prince R, Devine A, Dick I, et al. The effects of calcium supplementation (milk powder or tablets) and exercise on bone mineral density in postmenopausal women. J Bone Miner Res. 1995;10:1068–1075.

Spinach	93 mg
Swiss Chard	88 mg
Soybeans	60 mg
Leeks	52 mg
Broccoli	48 mg
Cauliflower	42 mg
Brussels Sprouts	36 mg

Producing meat and dairy products are bad for the environment because doing so leads to deforestation, species extinction, exorbitant use of resources like water and land, creates debilitating pollution, and emits greenhouse gasses, which contribute to climate change. The amount of water, grains, and soybeans it takes to feed animals requires significant amounts of water and land resources. These resources could be used instead to feed people in poor countries. Many of these countries are forced to grow crops to feed animals for profit instead of crops to feed people. Even fish farming has negative environmental impacts. It destroys precious sea life, like dolphins and sea turtles, pollutes the water with antibiotics and feces, and disturbs the ecosystem.

The pros of veganism outweigh the cons of meat and dairy consumption since veganism is better for the environment, your health, and the animals. People are far removed from the reality of how food gets from a farm or factory to the grocery store or to their plate. It's easy to order a burger at a restaurant or pick up the neatly packaged sausages and drumsticks at the grocery store without giving their processing or origins a second thought. If people could visit an industrial slaughterhouse and see the reality of the animals being harvested, killed, skinned, bleeding and chopped up, I wonder if they would still want to eat meat. I bet many people would be extremely turned off. Animals suffer unnecessarily in factory farms, and laboratories as they fall victim to extreme and unusual cruelty. Animal skins are needlessly used for fur and leather products (sometimes the animals are skinned alive and left to die). This burdens and angers my soul! By choosing products made without the use of animals, you are not supporting suffering. You don't have to support organizations that facilitate abuse. Being vegan is not just about health and beauty. It's also about compassion. Animals feel pain. Why do we have to exploit and hurt them? We don't. Knowing you are contributing to less animal suffering and less environmental damage might persuade you to decrease your meat and animal consumption or eradicate it altogether.

Not only are slaughterhouse practices horrible, but even so called humane farms are not that humane after all. Many people admit if they had to kill the animal, gut and clean it themselves, they would not be able to do it. The most recent available Census of Agriculture data shows that there were almost 95.5 million cows and calves in the United States in 2002.[44] There were also about 60.4 million hogs and pigs, each producing waste every day.[45] These numbers are making an epic impact on the environment. The amount of grain it takes to feed these animals could feed around 800 million people, and this type of farming is the leading consumer of water resources. Aside from environmental impact, meat is not so sanitary. Based on a consumer report examining the safety of ground beef, feces were found to be present in both conventional and organic beef. If that doesn't gross you out and shy you away from eating beef, then how about this? 458 pounds of both conventional and sustainable beef were tested for antibiotic resistant strains of bacteria; 18 percent of the conventional beef and 9 percent of the sustainable variety was found to contain drug resistant bacteria strains.[46] These crazy bacteria strains are found within chicken and pork, too. Animal farms become unsanitary grounds for these offenders to manifest themselves when animals get sick, die, and the others end up walking around or stepping on top of them.

Labels often are misleading. Eggs labeled as "cage free" lead us to believe that the chickens are running freely in grassy pastures, when they are still living in cruel conditions. The label "cage free" only means the chickens are not stacked up in cages, one upon another, and defecating on each other. Cage free chickens are often locked up in large, dark, overcrowded barns, sick and walking over the dead bodies of feathered friends who have not made it due to horrible living conditions. This is why if you choose to eat eggs, it's important to be conscious of their origin.

What is an egg anyway? It is an unfertilized egg meant to reproduce baby chicks. Women go through the same cycle every month, but chicken eggs are much larger. Does that sound appetizing to you, like something you want to eat? Male chicks aren't considered useful by the egg industry and its way of addressing this is to routinely shovel large batches of live chicks to their death by tossing them into a meat grinder. How is this even legal? Life does not be abused in this way and, therefore, eating and purchasing eggs becomes an issue of ethics. If you choose to consume eggs, purchase them from a reputable farm or a neighbor who keeps a chicken in the backyard to harvest eggs. You could even have your own chicken and name her Lucy.

---

44   USDA. (2002). Census of agriculture 2002: Cattle and calves. Retrieved August 27, 2012.

45   USDA. (2002). Census of agriculture 2002: Hogs and pigs. Retrieved August 27, 2012.

46   Rock, A., Consumer Report. (2015) How Safe is Your Ground Beef? Retrieved from www.consumerreports.org/cro/food/how-safe-is-your-ground-beef.htm

Eggs used to have a bad reputation because of their high cholesterol content and people were avoiding them or eating egg whites because they were concerned for health reasons. The American Heart Association now say eggs are okay because cholesterol has not been found to be associated with heart disease in some studies. Rather, saturated fat from dairy products and meats are the contributors to cardiovascular disease. Eggs are still high in cholesterol, containing around 237 milligrams per egg yolk, and nearly 70% fat, with 2 milligrams of saturated fat per egg.[47] Even though studies are showing eggs as safe for consumption, this is said to be in an amount of one egg per day, since a daily cholesterol limit has been set at around 300 mg.

Before we throw out the old notion that eggs are bad and accept the new idea that eggs are fine, let's dig a little deeper into some counter thoughts. Recent studies suggest that egg consumption is linked to heart disease because dietary cholesterol damages the arteries. Therefore, it would be wise to limit or forego eating eggs for preventative measures. Limiting cholesterol after a diagnosis is like quitting smoking after discovering you have lung cancer.[48] Even egg whites without the yolks or nonfat dairy products pose a threat because they are high in animal protein, which is linked to an increased risk of cancer. This is because animal protein increases production of an insulin-like growth factor that promotes proliferation of cancer cells.[49] An "egg-centered" breakfast is not the best choice, rather something plant-based is. Risk for diabetes was also shown to be associated with egg consumption, though more studies are necessary to explore why. It may be due to cholesterol raising blood glucose levels.[50]

Can cardiovascular disease and type 2 diabetes be reversed by following a vegan diet? The answers are yes and yes. Plant foods like smoothies, juices, and fruit are superior breakfast choices to eggs as they are related to lower rates of cardiovascular disease and overall lower mortality. Many of our favorite desserts use eggs, and so do a lot of the Keto, Paleo, and other low carb diets (they use a lot). Don't worry if you love to bake! Delicious desserts, breads, cakes, cookies, and pancakes can all be made with a variety of whole food, plant-based egg alternatives.

We can make the choice to collectively address issues of ethics and health through how we eat and the products we purchase. People who care about the wellbeing of others and the pres-

47   Spence JD, Jenkins DJ, Davignon J. Dietary cholesterol and egg yolks: not for patients at risk of vascular disease. Can J Cardiol. 2010;26:336-339.
48   Spence JD, Jenkins DJ, Davignon J. Dietary cholesterol and egg yolks: not for patients at risk of vascular disease. Can J Cardiol. 2010;26:336-339.
49   Fuhrman, J. (2004-2018). Animal Protein is Linked to an Increased Risk of Cancer. Retrieved from https://www.drfuhrman.com/learn/library/articles/2/animal-protein-is-linked-to-increased-risk-of-cancer
50   Li Y, Zhou C, Zhou X, Li L. Egg consumption and risk of cardiovascular diseases and diabetes: a meta-analysis. Atherosclerosis. 2013;229:524-530.

ervation of the environment could consider a more plant-based way of life—if not completely, then mostly. This would increase the available number of crops that could feed people globally, decrease pollution, and save water and energy. Plant-based living is a movement on the rise, reawakened as the concept has been around for years. Impacts of an increase in vegan living would minimize the clearing of rainforests, and grains that would normally feed livestock could be exported to impoverished countries.

Animals are raised and slaughtered unethically and unjustly. Ask yourself if killing animals is ethical to you in the first place. Any being with a nervous system feels pain and suffering, and why should humans be allowed to exploit, abuse, and murder innocent living beings at the expense of a burger, milkshake, or hot wing? It is not okay to use and abuse them for profit, especially for an industry culminating sickness and disease. It's just not necessary, especially when there are so many delicious vegan foods that taste even better than their cruel counterpart. According to Steve Cockerham, a USDA inspector at Nebraska slaughterhouses, and former USDA veterinarian, Lester Friedlander, some U.S. slaughterhouses routinely skin live cattle and immerse squealing pigs in scalding water. People in the vegan community choose to live the lifestyle for different reasons: some of them ethical, some environmental, for health reasons, beauty reasons, or all the above. I encourage you to become aware and have compassion.

Social justice is also an issue at hand when it comes to producing animals for food. Large animal farms, particularly pig and chicken farms in North Carolina, for example, produce insurmountable amounts of waste that is disposed of near and around African American and Latino homes.[51] This unwanted burden is damaging their communities and waterways as they become polluted. Fish die as a result, and people are afraid to drink water from local wells. Residents in these North Carolina communities feel depressed and appalled at the stench coming from the farms. The United States Government and Accountability office published that, in 2002, North Carolina ran through 7.5 million pigs, producing 15.5 million tons of waste.[52] Not only is the waste a concern, but toxic chemicals become a problem because they are in the grass and animal feed as genetically modified soy, corn, and wheat. When humans eat the animals, they ingest cancer-causing poisons.

These are many reasons to switch to a plant-based diet or at least drastically cut back on animal product consumption. What we eat and drink becomes us and reflects in our energy and well-being. If we are eating foods that come from sick and abused factory farms, that negative food energy

51　Fine, E., Hellerstein & K. (2017) A Million Tons of Feces and Unbearable Stench: Life Near Industrial Pig Farms. Retrieved from https://www.drfuhrman.com/learn/library/articles/2/animal-protein-is-linked-to-increased-risk-of-cancer
52　http://www.gao.gov/new.items/d08944.pdf

could affect our health and wellbeing, aside from the harmful impacts animal production has on the environment and surrounding communities. It's not fair to the living and breathing animals nor the people who suffer from exposure to animal waste pollution. Foods from the earth, like fruits, vegetables, beans, nuts, and seeds, support every aspect of energy, beauty, and health. If we make the choice to eat vegan or plant-based, we support ourselves, avoid needless suffering, and spare the environment.

CHAPTER 8
DON'T PANIC!
CHOOSE ORGANIC

It is universally known that fruits and vegetables are good for us. Unfortunately, not all fruits and vegetables are created equal. By now, you have heard about organic foods and may be wondering why you should spend more money on organic food opposed to the more affordable non-organic foods. What does organic mean exactly? Certified organic labeling means 95% of the labeled product must be organic and grown in soil not containing synthetic fertilizers and pesticides. The demand for organic foods has increased and people are becoming more aware of what is good for them. There is a myriad of reasons why organic foods are the best for us. In this chapter, we will be looking at the reasons why organic is a better choice than conventional foods. Conventional food practices are opposite to organic practices and rely on chemicals, hormones, antibiotics, and GMOs to produce food.

Conventional produce is sprayed with pesticides to kill pests and is often genetically modified, which poses potential health risks. Pesticides are linked to cancer, attention deficit disorder, attention deficit hyperactivity disorder, birth defects, and more. In 1993, an Agricultural Health Study was conducted by the National Cancer Institute to examine the effects of agricultural exposures to pesticides on farm workers and the surrounding communities. Findings about the relationship between cancer rates of farmers and agricultural workers compared to people outside of that job arena were significant. "Farming communities have higher rates of leukemia, non-Hodgkin lymphoma, multiple myeloma, and soft tissue sarcoma, as well as cancers of the skin, lip, stomach, brain, and prostate." The Agricultural Health Study also revealed some eye-opening information. Findings concluded that people exposed to the weed killer imazethapyr have increased risks of bladder cancer and colon cancer. People with the highest cumulative lifetime exposure had more than twice the risk (137% increase in risk) of developing bladder cancer compared with those who had no exposure to the chemical. Since 1989, it has been one of the most commonly used herbicides for killing weeds in soybean, dry bean, alfalfa, and other crop fields.[53]

---

53   Agricultural Health Study, National Cancer Institute, www.cancer.gov/about-cancer/causes-prevention/risk/ahs-fact-sheet#q1

Chemicals created to kill weeds, insects, and small animals are being sprayed on and infused into foods via conventional farming practices and genetic modification. Consumers beware that these poisons don't just affect pests, they affect people as well. Although publications also state that more research is needed to become conclusive on the specific cause, this information is enough to cause a stir of concern about safety and the use of pesticides. The documentary "The Human Experiment" released in 2013 educates viewers about the rise in birth defects, autism, learning disabilities, infertility, cancer, and questions them being linked to pesticides and other environmental toxins. I recommend watching it as this movie is informative and thought provoking.

Pesticide consumption through food should be avoided whenever possible. How is this done? First, being educated about the risks are important because knowledge is power and leads to change. The process starts at home with parent education and it is essential to get more schools on board with proper nutrition education for children and parents. This is big. Seek out organic produce whenever you can. Purchasing produce from farmer's markets is the best because you find the freshest and tastiest organic produce. A lot of the non-organic produce at farmer's markets is usually not sprayed with pesticides as well.

The American Academy of Environmental Medicine urges doctors to tell patients to eat non-GMO foods. These doctors are citing animal studies that have shown organ damage, gastrointestinal and immune system disorders, accelerated aging, and infertility linked to eating GMO foods. Human studies are showing how GM food can leave material behind inside of us, and toxic insecticide produced by GM corn was found in the blood of pregnant women and unborn fetuses.[54] With disease and cancer rates at an all-time high and on the rise, let us think about how genetically modified food is affecting humanity. The largely produced GM crops are wheat, corn, and soy, which are found in nearly every processed food product and even foods that are marketed wisely to appear as "healthy." People eat GM processed foods every day and think nothing of it. Genetically modified foods were introduced in 1996 and, since then, the percentage of Americans with three or more chronic illnesses has jumped from 7% to 13%, food allergies have risen tremendously, rates of autism, reproductive disorders and digestive problems have increased as well.[55] Unfortunately, there is not enough research to confirm that GMOs are directly to blame, but with what we DO know, it is not a far cry to assume that they could have something to do with it.

This is all food for thought and why I choose non-GMO foods whenever possible. More

54   Smith, Jeffery, Responsibletechnology.org 10 Reasons to Avoid GMOs
55   Smith, Jeffrey, Responsibletechnology.org, 10 Reasons to Avoid GMOs

and more children are suffering from ADHD than ever before, which leads to learning difficulties and disruptive behavior. Why is this? An article published in the journal of pediatrics found a direct link to pesticides and ADHD. It is stated that "the toxins affect the nervous system, which is how pests are killed." Researchers measured the levels of pesticide byproducts in the urine of 1,139 children from across the United States. Children with above-average levels of one common byproduct had roughly twice the odds of getting a diagnosis of ADHD.[56] Children are the most sensitive to chemicals, which is alarming because the food they eat in school is not organic, most likely genetically modified, and low quality meat is often used for meals. While California schools are making improvements to their lunch programs, they need continued improvement. Schools could offer foods that are safer for children to eat, that will promote learning from the standpoint that they are not GM and are organic, whole foods at best (not processed). Some school have gardens on site and use that food for school meals. This not only is healthier, but students could get involved and learn more about the process of growing food while building a sense of community.

Globally, genetically modified foods are said to provide food to feed the impoverished and combat famine now and in the future. Is this truly the answer to these problems? Perhaps not. Genetically modified organisms were developed in the 1980s for agricultural purposes like pest control, drought resistance, herbicide tolerance, disease resistance, and enhanced nutritional profiling. The process of genetically modifying crops allows the traits of plants to be changed by transferring genetic information from one source to another. Biotechnology companies like Monsanto, Dupont, Dow, and Syngenta create genetically modified seeds. Monsanto monopolizes this arena. These companies claim that producing food this way will provide benefits to global world issues like hunger and nutrition problems. The answers to these issues lay more in allocating resources used for factory farming, thus dedicating them to resolving world hunger rather than creating produce in the lab, thus more pest resistant foods and crops. This would be far more effective than producing animals for food consumption.

Many European countries have been able to do away with GMO foods because they have demanded labeling of such foods. The effect of labeling caused a decrease in GMO consumption, and the demand for non-GMO foods increased through supply and demand. In 2010, when an earthquake devastated much of Haiti, Monsanto donated pesticides, hybrid seeds, and fertilizers to assist the grief-stricken nation in rehabilitating its food supply. Haiti's Ministry of Agriculture rejected the donation of GMO Roundup seeds, and thousands of farmers protested and burned hybrid corn seeds, rejecting any further shipments. Haitian leaders are invested in preserving their agriculture, native

56   CNN.com, Study ADHD Linked to Pesticide Exposure

biodiversity, and environmental integrity true to Mother Earth.

Even though many countries have taken a stance against GMO food production due to its risks and dangers, America hasn't. About thirty-seven countries have already banned GMO crop cultivation. Some of them include Algeria (since 2000), Madagascar (since 2002), Turkey, Switzerland, Italy, Russia, Greece, Bulgaria, Ecuador, France, Peru, Venezuela, and Saudi Arabia.[57] Take a stand against GMO foods by purchasing non-GMO foods (a.k.a. organic). There is a battle in efforts to prove scientifically that GMOs are, in fact, harmful. New studies are showing their negative impacts, whereas other published studies show no harmful effects of GMOs to humans or animals.[58] On the other hand, one study concluded that GM foods are related to gluten related disorders, celiac, and autoimmune disorders. Gilles-Eric Séralini lead a scientific study for the Food and Chemical Toxicology journal. This study correlated rat tumors and GM corn. Scientists scorned the article for not using a large enough number of animals in the study. Though the article was retracted, many scientists disagree with that decision. I find it interesting that the Food and Chemical Toxicology Journal would dismiss these findings and forcibly retract the article. Appointed editor and biologists affiliated with this decision just happens to have worked for Monsanto for seven years. The study found that rats fed for two years with Monsanto's glyphosate-resistant NK603 maize (corn) developed many more tumors and died earlier than controls. It also found that the rats developed tumors when glyphosate (Roundup), the herbicide used with GM maize, was added to their drinking water.[59] Other GM red flags include their relatedness to birth defects, autism, Parkinson's, Alzheimer's, and breast cancer by way of a toxin called glyphosate.[60]

With our food supply being modified genetically, our bodies are essentially ingesting new food. Wheat, corn, and soy are not the same as they were a hundred years ago (untampered with and designed by nature). Even the animals people eat are consuming genetically modified feed, so meat is different as well. Our bodies are not designed to break down chemically altered, processed fats or partially hydrogenated oils, for example. Neither are they accustomed to the evolution of genetically modified food.

Let's face it. Organic food generally costs more, and processed food is viewed as being cheaper. While eating organic is possible for people on a tight budget, people who cannot afford to

57   http://sustainablepulse.com/2015/10/22/gm-crops-now-banned-in-36-countries-worldwide-sustainable-pulse-research/#.WPu45t-Lyu02

58   Snell, C., Bernheim, A.,Berge, J.B., Kuntz, M., Pascal, G., Paris, A., Ricroch., Assessment of the Health Impact of GM Plant Diets in Long Term, and Multigenerational Animal Feeding Trials. Food and Chemical Toxicology. (2012) 1134-1148.

59   Casassus, B., (2013) Study linking GM maize to rat tumors is retracted. Retrieved from https://www.nature.com/news/study-linking-gm-maize-to-rat-tumours-is-retracted-1.14268

60   Walia, A. (2014)10 Scientific Studies Proving GMOs Can be Harmful to Human Health. Retrieved from https://www.rt.com/usa/gmo-gluten-sensitivity-trigger-343/

spend more on food are more likely to choose foods that could potentially make them sick. I spend a good chunk of change monthly on organic produce, which I view as an investment in my health. I notice the prices are higher than conventional produce, and I feel privileged to eat the way I do. Why does organic produce have inflated costs? A salad at a fast food restaurant costs more than a burger. Something is wrong with that picture. If governing officials would provide support to organic farmers instead of subsidizing commercial wheat, corn, and soy crops for the companies producing processed foods, then perhaps organic food would be accessible to more people who are concerned about the cost. It is obvious to see that eating a diet high in fruits and vegetables could easily add up in one's budget. This is a problem because, in many cases, organic food does cost more. A conventional head of celery costs $0.99 compared to $2.99 for organic celery in a grocery store.

Something needs to be done about this on a governmental level. Organic farmers need support through government subsidizing to keep costs down, and more people buying organic will create cost minimization. Shop the farmer's markets for produce and bulk sections at the grocery stores. If you go at closing time, farmer's market vendors will discount the produce greatly and you can wheel and deal. As a vegan, you are not buying expensive meat, dairy products, and fish, so you might be able to more easily afford to spend a few extra dollars on produce. Despite this, there are ways to make a clean way of eating affordable; even as affordable as buying processed or convenience food. If you are not buying everything organic but have eliminated processed foods and have switched to whole plant foods, that is a big step in the right direction.

Here and now, in this increasingly complex food culture, there is more to consider when it comes to eating food, even food that appears to be healthy. It's as if we must navigate through a web of conflicting dietary advice to choose the right foods because labeling is deceiving. Eating is undeniably simple when you stick to unaltered, chemical-free, natural food. Well-meaning consumers are led to believe they are buying something healthy due to misleading food labels. For example, many bread and cereal products are advertised as whole grain when, in fact, they are not. It is best to avoid packaged foods and stick to unprocessed whole foods straight from nature. If you have kids, set an example by modeling how to eat, and educate them about why you are making good food choices. More children would be attracted to eating fruits and vegetables if they were marketed and advertised to in popular culture with cartoon characters and celebrity promotions in the same way processed, sugary cereals, popular soft drinks, and fast food chains are. We need leaders in the advertising industry and celebrities to take part in helping make the shift towards glamorizing fruits and vegetables.

Not only is organic food safer to consume, but the taste of organic produce as compared to non-organic is incomparable. Organic produce delivers such great flavor that when you experience the difference, you will become hooked and possibly turn into somewhat of a food snob. When you have non-organic produce, you might wonder why you wasted your money on flavorless produce laced with toxic compounds designed to kill bugs. It just doesn't taste the same, and what will that poison do to your body? Once people become educated about food and its production, I believe they will make better decisions for themselves and their families. The larger problem at hand rests in the politics of food.

Is anybody surprised that the largest company of genetically modified foods and heavily laden crops has totally monopolized the farming industry and funds many politicians who make decisions about food production in America? The FDA also allows for chemicals, like compounds used in paint thinner, to mimic the cherry flavor you taste in artificially flavored cherry ice cream. Do you think you should trust the government or the FDA, and do you want to eat that stuff?

There are several widespread chemicals and practices that have been banned in Europe that are still allowed under FDA regulation in America. For example, a UK study found a correlation between artificial food colors, additives, and ADHD in children aged 3 years and 8-9 years of age.[61] Europe at large labels and warns consumers of the adverse effects on behavior and the UK has banned them altogether. The United States has done nothing of the sort. Children eat and drink these chemicals daily. It is mind boggling that chemicals like bread conditioner potassium bromate (used to increase dough strength and flexibility) was banned in the European Union, China, Canada, and Brazil, but not in America. Unfortunately, consumers cannot trust the government or the healthcare system when it comes to safe product distribution, and one must take responsibility for their own health.

Who would you rather pay? The farmer or the doctor? Begin to look at food as preventative medicine that will keep you well instead of something to just please the senses or fill voids. Having said that, as you crowd out junk foods, animal fat, salt, and sugar, and begin replacing them with whole, fresh foods, your taste buds will adjust to appreciate the natural flavor in foods. You will begin to crave healthy foods and your taste buds will not be disappointed by many of the fantastic vegan recipes in this book and out there in the world. I am amazed daily at the delicious alternatives to conventional foods. Not only is it fun to try new vegan foods, but many of my meat-eating friends and relatives love the foods I make and share with love from my kitchen.

61   McCann D1, Barrett A, Cooper A, Crumpler D, Dalen L, Grimshaw K, Kitchin E, Lok K, Porteous L, Prince E, Sonuga-Barke E, Warner JO, Stevenson J.Food, Additives and hyperactive behaviour in 3-year-old and 8/9-year-old children in the community, https://www.ncbi.nlm.nih.gov/pubmed/17825405

Eating local means you are supporting local farmers by purchasing your fruits and vegetables at the farmer's market or from vendors that carry foods grown close to home. Farmer's markets sell produce that is in season and eating in season supports the body's efforts to adapt to the environment. Eating fruit in season works to keep the body cool in the summertime, whereas eating foods harvested in the winter, like squash, work to keep the body warm. Seasonal eating also lessens the carbon footprint left by transporting foods across the globe. These foods are the freshest and taste great.

Speaking of eating local, you can't get much more local than having your own garden. Growing your own food is a trend, and it's one I am looking forward to in the future. Purchasing local produce makes a difference because many of these farmers do not use pesticides. Produce harvested early from foreign countries must be shipped from hundreds and thousands of miles away, which requires a great deal of fossil fuel consumption. Conventional produce found in supermarkets is usually covered with a protective wax to ensure freshness, improve the appearance, prevent molding, and reduce the likelihood of contamination. Apples, for example, might have a shelf life of a couple of years. This does not sound appealing, no pun intended, but the FDA has deemed the waxes safe for human consumption.

Knowing which conventional fruits and vegetables are safest to eat is a step in the right direction and can help defer the cost of organic eating. This means you can pick and choose the items you need to buy organic and the items for which it isn't as important to buy organic. A resource known as the "Dirty Dozen and Clean 15" provides a guide to follow for safe and wise produce consumption. Below, I provide a list of fruits and vegetables (reaching past the clean 15) in order from the most laden with pesticides to the least. You want to buy the first fifteen items organic since they contain the most pesticides, especially porous produce like strawberries because they easily soak in the elements. The items towards the end of the list are safer to eat conventionally since they contain lesser amounts of pesticides. Foods with thick skin like bananas, mangoes, and avocados are safer to eat commercially as well since the skins are not consumed or as porous. The organic varieties taste better, and are grown in higher quality soil which, in turn, lends to the quality of the food. Buying organic food also safeguards you from the dangers of consuming genetically modified organisms (GMOs).

Conventional Produce List

(in order from most pesticide sprayed to least: WORST TO BEST [62])

1. Strawberries
2. Apples
3. Nectarines
4. Peaches
5. Celery
6. Grapes
7. Cherries
8. Spinach
9. Tomatoes
10. Sweet Bell Peppers
11. Cherry Tomatoes
12. Cucumbers
13. Imported Snap Peas
14. Domestic Blueberries
15. Potatoes
16. Hot Peppers
17. Lettuce
18. Kale/Collard Greens
19. Imported Blueberries
20. Green Beans
21. Plums
22. Pears
23. Raspberries
24. Carrots
25. Winter Squash
26. Tangerines
27. Summer Squash
28. Domestic Snap Peas
29. Green Onions
30. Bananas
31. Oranges
32. Watermelon
33. Broccoli
34. Sweet Potatoes
35. Mushrooms
36. Cauliflower
37. Grapefruit
38. Honeydew
39. Eggplant
40. Kiwi
41. Papayas
42. Mangos
43. Asparagus
44. Onions
45. Frozen Sweet Peas
46. Cabbage
47. Pineapple
48. Sweet Corn
49. Avocados

The PLU code, known as the Price Lookup Code, is another way to decipher between differ-ent kinds of produce. This code can be found on the stickers adhered to fruits and vegetables. If the code has four digits and begins with a 4, then it was grown conventionally and with pesticides (for example, 4011). If the code begins with an 8 and has five digits, then it is genetically modified (for example, 84011). Produce starting with a 9 (for example, 94011) is organic and cannot be genetically modified since organic produce does not practice the use of GMOs. If you buy non-organic produce, remember to wash it well with a produce wash. You can purchase a produce wash or make one at home. Making your own is an inexpensive and easy way to clean your fruits and vegetables.

Do-it-Yourself Fruit and Vegetable Wash

1. Fill a large bowl or sink with water.

2. Then add 1 cup of white vinegar and mix it around.

3. Add in your produce and let it soak for about 10 minutes.

4. Give your produce a final rinse to wash off the vinegar water.

After you soak the produce, you should notice that the water is dirty since it has removed the junk from your produce. This will help your fruit stay fresh longer as well.

Food is evolving and changing faster than our bodies can adapt. How can our systems rec-ognize these chemical, toxic, and foreign compounds (GM foods)? What are the cancer and disease rates in America telling us? These rates keep increasing and are expected to continue to do so. Food is easy, yet it has become complicated. It's time to get back to the basics—the real basics. Eat natural, chemical-free, non-GMO food. An apple is no longer an apple; it's either a waxed, bland, Roundup laced, apple grown in chemical fertilizer, denatured soil apple, or it's an organic, tasty, crisp, and nutri-tious apple. Our bodies need real food to thrive.

CHAPTER 9
7 SHADES OF VEGAN

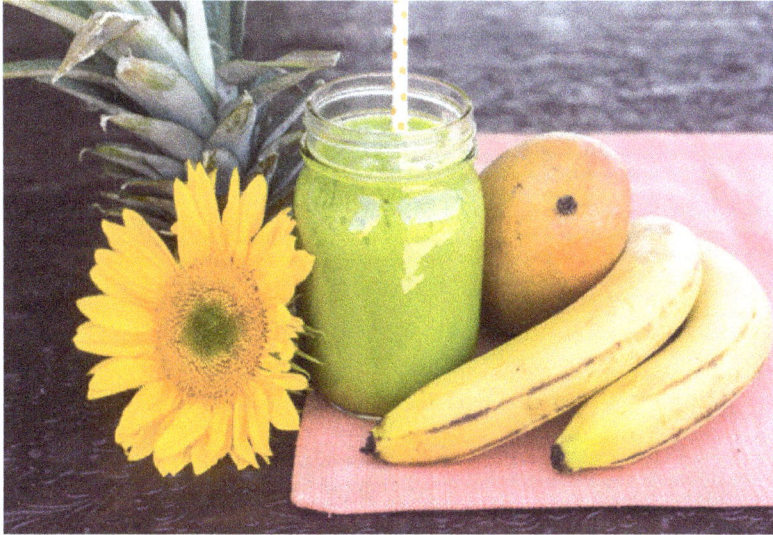

Aside from ethical reasons, your health is big reason to go vegan and there are different ways to go about it. This section shares some of the different styles and options of vegan. Hopefully this will help you to find the shade or shades that work best for you! When I was a kid in elementary school, Jump Rope for Heart was (and still is) a fundraising event for the American Heart Association. Us kids would go out onto the playground and jump rope our brains out, while we had fun getting heart healthy exercise. Kids today are still doing this! Heart disease is the number one killer in America. According to Doctor T. Colin Campbell, almost 2,000 Americans will die from this disease every twenty-four hours. In his book, *The China Study,* Campbell and other renowned doctors discuss how a whole foods, plant-based diet reverses heart disease and saves lives, as they have witnessed this through application and studies with patients.[63] Doctor Neal Barnard, in his research efforts and

---

63   Campbell, T.C., & Campbell, T.M., (2006) The China Study, Dallas, TX: Books.

education in association with the Physicians Committee for Responsible Medicine, also reports the benefits of a vegan diet to manage weight, diabetes, cholesterol, migraines, heart disease and more.[64]

Going deeper, I have experienced a spiritual awakening as well as my own beautiful awakening that has led me to express love and gratitude for not just people, but for animals. I am inspired by the gifts of nature such as fruits, vegetables, plants, and the ocean. I wish for the planet to be at peace, and for animals to experience freedom. Aside from God, first and foremost, raw veganism has allowed me to find myself, heal physically, connect spiritually and become stronger in my convictions. Through my transition, I focused on my purpose and talents. I learned about acceptance and that being uniquely different is okay. Many times, I find myself marching to the beat of my own drum and have had to be honest and advocate for my choices and beliefs. I embrace being different because I can lead others, and would rather stand out in a crowd than blend in. It took me many years in my life before I could confidently do that, and it feels empowering. It once felt embarrassing and shameful (in the beginning when friends and relatives did not understand or accept my lifestyle choices), but this awakening is due to a mental and physical cleansing and rebuilding of the body.

Being vegan does wonders for your physical fitness and I crave movement most days. Even on the days when I am exhausted and want to do nothing, I find it difficult to be sedentary. Most of all, I don't have to overdo it to get muscle tone and stay slender because plants are full of fiber, water and nutrients, so my body is satisfied with appropriate amounts of food and nutrition. When people eat empty calories or food low in nutrition, they may be eating large amounts but still feel hungry because their bodies are not getting the nutrients it needs. This is a recipe for obesity. My appetite opened when I became vegan, and I could still enjoy a wide array of foods to satisfy cravings. This allows me to have a positive relationship with food and stay off the hamster wheel of food addiction and remorse. I don't feel restricted and I love to eat. I can eat as much as I need to and I don't have to think much about it. Knowing that what I'm eating is going to digest well and nourish my body without negative affects gives me peace of mind to focus on other important aspects of life.

Vegans take pride in knowing their food choices benefit humanity and do not support animal cruelty while sparing the environment of unnecessary waste and degradation. Being more conscious and less confused about mainstream media and the latest diet fads has liberated me to unplug from the chatter and be enlightened by a more minimalist approach to life. With strength and energy gained from fruits and vegetables, the body becomes more ageless and vibrant. Do yourself a favor,

64   Physicians Committee for Responsible Medicine. Cholesterol and Heart Disease. Retrieved from http://www.pcrm.org/health/health-topics/cholesterol-and-heart-disease

spare some animals, the environment, have more energy, and look younger as well. You have every-thing to gain.

Maybe you don't know where to start. What will you do when you miss all the old foods you will be leaving behind? You may be wondering about what to eat, how to prepare such foods, and how to get enough of the macro and micro nutrients like protein, iron, and calcium. If you think about it, most animals people eat get their nutrition from plants. Plants are primary sources of nutrition from the soil, water, and sun. If a cow, gorilla, or rhinoceros can live and be strong by eating only plants, so can you. Animals are a secondary source of protein.

Let's talk about how to adopt a whole food, plant-based lifestyle without shocking your body and mind. There will be a transitionary period, so take it slowly and take your time. I was on a back and forth journey for over ten years before I made the decision to go all in. Initially, I just wanted to experience better health and healing. Now, I choose to stick to it for ethical reasons. It feels amazing to live consciously, eating food that loves you back. Start with small changes, like replacing breakfast and lunch with healthy vegan meals and make dinner as usual. Use smaller amounts of animal prod-ucts and eventually replace them all with your favorite plant-based alternatives. Your taste buds will shift to crave healthy foods over time. Remain flexible and remember the goal is not perfection. The vegan lifestyle is not about limiting yourself or dieting in any way. Transitioning is as easy or difficult as you choose it to be. Our approach to what we experience in life has meaning based on the thoughts we give it. If we think something is difficult or impossible, then it is. On the other hand, if we think something is more easily achievable and fun, then it is. Mindset is key. I would rather experience a temporary detox or cleanse than a life full of undesirable health.

Think about what has attracted you to this lifestyle and write down what you want to get out of it. Your journey can be taken in baby steps or strides. Imagine crowding out meat and dairy with delicious fruits, vegetables, nuts, and seeds combined in recipes that will satisfy all your cravings and nutritional needs. The alternatives are plentiful, and there really is a way to make this work for you if you so desire. You are opening yourself up to magic and freedom that you can only experience once you step outside the box of conventional thinking and eating. A vegan lifestyle increases your lifes-pan. Vegetarians are known to live five years longer and vegans are known to live seven years longer than the average person on a standard American diet.

Diet is not something we should treat dogmatically or have an all or nothing mentality with. Remain flexible, allowing yourself some wiggle room to experiment or fail when discovering what works for you. At times, we must slip into and experience old habits to appreciate what we now have and stay on track. Some people go vegan overnight because they want to lose weight and look more beautiful, but that may not be enough to anchor your convictions for giving up animal products. Others start out as vegetarians and go back and forth between eating meat, fish, and dairy products for some time before they finally make the change for good. People feel and see the difference in themselves when they give up animal products and eat plants! They want to continue because they are loving it. Eating a plant-based diet really shifts everything for the better, and once people learn the truth about the horrors of the meat and dairy industry, hearts will be impacted and lasting change can occur.

Vegan meals done right are delicious and filling. After trying them, you may find that you do not miss your former style of eating, or you will want to incorporate more plant-based foods into your diet. Depending on where you live, there are vegan options almost anywhere you go. Restaurants are offering more healthy alternatives for customers and the movement is growing. I have been able to make this way of eating manageable in any situation, whether it has been while traveling, at work, on the go, at social gatherings, or at holiday affairs.

Navigating New Dietary Choices

Food does more than just fuel our bodies. It's something that, for many, serves emotional needs and connects people socially. People fall into patterns of emotional eating and this is where the term "comfort food" stems from. We may associate happiness with eating something special, use food as a reward mechanism, eat when we're sad, stressed out, or use food to cope with a lack of intimacy or loneliness.

People have trouble standing by their dietary choices due to emotional attachments to food and may struggle with giving up certain things for social reasons. They do not want to draw attention to themselves for being different or not eating how everybody else eats, especially at social and family gatherings. Perhaps they feel like they are hurting someone's feelings by not eating food that was especially prepared for an occasion. I can remember many times feeling like the odd ball out because I was making different food choices, and I think it has taken my poor father a long time to get over the fact that I'm not eating his prized prepared dishes any longer. It used to make me sad sometimes, as if I was rejecting my friends or family for not eating the familiar foods that were served. In the beginning, those feelings were challenging, however, over time, I learned to use them as opportunities to connect with people in other ways besides through food. For example, if I felt sad about not eating my dad's chicken, instead, I could spend time with him talking during dinner and then let him know that I love him. During the holidays, a vegan might feel a sense of missing out or disconnectedness because of the food separation. Food is not what matters most when it comes to relationships and social interactions. Relationships are about love, conversation, connection, giving and receiving. These are the things I focus on at social gatherings now as opposed to what I'm not eating.

When I attend food related social gatherings, I make food and bring it to share. I focus on spending time with the people I love while we have fun making new memories. That's really what it's all about. If anybody feels threatened or upset by the fact that you no longer eat foods you once did, it's not your problem, and that is okay. Love and accept yourself. It's not your job to make everybody happy. People should accept you for who you are no matter what you eat. Over time, you will inspire people by living a healthy lifestyle and they will see how you look and feel better. The proof is in the pudding. Just think about how good it would feel to not have to depend on medications, looking five to ten years younger than you are, and having as much energy as people half your age. There are many variations or ways to go vegan within the paradigm, and I'd like to present seven different styles of eating to consider when choosing or experimenting with the vegan lifestyle. Let's explore the 7 Shades of Vegan.

Shade 1 - The Original Vegan Diet

The term "vegan" stands for excluding all animal products including honey, gelatin, meat, and dairy products. The original vegan diet includes soy foods, wheat products, grains, beans, fruits, nuts, seeds, legumes, vegetables, and anything else considered vegan for that matter. Traditional vegan foods include things like wheat bread, seitan (wheat gluten made as a meat alternative), alternative cheeses, vegan pizzas, tofu, oatmeal, and faux meats that imitate things like chicken, steak, and even seafood. Having these options to replace familiar foods can be quite helpful for people who can tolerate soy and gluten and are just transitioning to the lifestyle. Fake meats are usually made of wheat gluten or soy and are somewhat of a novelty because you can get things like "chicken nuggets" and "buffalo wings." They look and taste much like the real thing, except they are made from plant-based products instead of meat. The problem is wheat and soy are both ingredients high on the list of food allergens, and they can lead to digestive discomfort and skin issues. Plus, they are processed. People who are newly transitioning to the diet may find these foods helpful to have as an option if they miss meat and dairy foods, but should not be overeaten. I don't think processed fake meats are healthy foods.

If you want to go vegan in an effortless way, start by finding replacements for the animal products you normally use like meat, eggs, milk, and honey. It's easy to replace those ingredients. For example, use maple syrup instead of honey, mushrooms or beans instead of meat, and flax meal "eggs" instead of eggs. Find your favorite type of plant-based milk like hemp, almond, or coconut to replace cow's milk. If you miss foods like cheese, pizza, or cheesecake, try some of the soy-free vegan versions in moderation.

Eating at restaurants is easy, too! I see many vegan options at restaurants and you can always ask the server to modify a dish for you. I have eaten out at some of the fanciest non-vegan restaurants as a raw-vegan and the kitchen staff is always able to put something together for me, like a large salad with plenty of fresh vegetables from the menu with avocado. Dressing might be salsa, lemon, oil and vinegar, or a simple vinaigrette. Don't be embarrassed to ask for modifications. You only live once, and why not? It's better to socialize sometimes and not be tied down to only eating at home.

I do prefer food I prepare at home in my kitchen, and once you get the hang of it, you will too! You can control the ingredients and put love energy into the food you make. When I first heard that idea, I thought, "Put love into it? That's weird." After pondering the concept, I decided to give it a try. You know what? It works. The food tastes great and people will take notice. To do this, raise your consciousness when you begin to prepare food. You must slow down, clean the space, and remember why you're doing it and choose to feel the love and positive energy vibes. Even when I'm tired or not in the mood, I tap into the feeling of love and envision it going into the food, appreciating the nourishment, energy, health, and beauty it will give me. That's motivation to put out the effort it takes to shop for and prepare food at home 24/7. I imagine the great way I will feel because of meal prep and juicing. It's worthwhile work, a MUST, and you will thank yourself for these efforts. To ease the need to constantly be at the grocery store, stocking up on produce and other foods, I have fresh, local, and organic produce delivered to my doorstep once a week through an online service. I get to choose what goes in my box and I love it because I always have something on-hand to work with. I also order many of the other products I use online. I get free shipping and my box comes within a few days. This makes food prep effortless, simple, and fun.

Keeping food as close to nature as possible is the goal. Vegan meals can be versatile, even without the fake meats. With the right dressings and sauces, you can enjoy many different vegetables eaten raw, steamed, roasted, or stir-fried with a variety of legumes, grains, nuts, seeds, baked squashes, and potatoes. Pastas are now made from many other ingredients besides wheat, like brown rice, lentils, quinoa, and black beans. An original vegan eats any and everything vegan under the sun in a healthy and balanced way.

The vegan food pyramid illustrates a healthful and balanced guide of what to eat. A vegan diet is easy and doable for many people once you know what the alternatives are. A typical day might include oatmeal and fruit for breakfast, soup, salad, and crackers for lunch, apples with almond butter for a snack, and stir-fried veggies with brown rice and tempeh for dinner. Dessert could be vegan versions of dark chocolate or fudge brownies. Meal options are endless, as you could also have vegan versions of curries, Thai food, pastas, pizza, wraps, salads, and more. Since the foods are high in fiber and lighter than their animal counterparts, you get to eat more and until you are full. Eat more and still look amazing? Yes, please.

There is no need for deprivation or calorie counting. I stopped counting calories years ago. Who has time for that? You don't, and you don't need to. Discovering new fruits or veggie meals is exciting and trying new vegan restaurants is fun. Finding recipes you enjoy is key, and having support along the way is essential to any successful lifestyle outcome.

Shade 2 - The Grain-Free Vegan

Have you tried going vegan and you're still not feeling as good as you think you should? Do you still suffer from poor digestion, brain fog, skin issues, or fatigue? There are valid reasons to include grains in one's diet but, on the flip side, there are just as many reasons to avoid eating grains. Grains include foods like wheat, millet, corn, rice, barley, oats, sorghum, spelt, rye, bulgur, and buckwheat. Grains are affordable, nutritious, full of fiber, and filling, however, if inflammation and digestion are not under control in the body, they could be doing more harm than good. Plenty of doctors and nutritionists recommend grains as part of a healthy vegan diet, and they are not necessarily wrong. There are many conflicting dietary opinions and what works for one person may not work for another. You must decide for yourself what is best.

The trend of going grain-free has become popular thanks to the paleo diet, and people are getting results. If you don't want to consume animal products, you can still maintain a healthy, plant-based, grain-free diet. Try switching to a grain-free regimen for four to six weeks to see the difference it makes in how you feel. Then you can introduce one grain at a time to see which ones you can tolerate, if any. Examine how your body reacts to specific grains and experiment with using different grain free alternatives to replace grains in your diet.

As a grain-free vegan, you can include legumes, nuts, and seeds as a part of your diet. Foods like beans, quinoa, cassava, flax, nut flours, and chia fill the nutrition gaps where grains are absent. The possibilities of dishes and food combinations are endless, and if you feel amazing by excluding grains from your diet, then perhaps you have struck gold with this shade of vegan. Focus on the foods you can eat instead of what you are not eating and, once again, find new and delicious recipes you enjoy.

If you are going to shun grains while maintaining a vegan diet, you should do it very intentionally to ensure a variety of nutrition is attained for nourishment. You may be thinking, *What is there left to eat?* There is a whole lot, including raw and cooked foods, such as sweet potatoes, sea vegetables, squashes, sprouts, coconuts, root vegetables, seeds, nuts, nut butters, quinoa, and wild black rice. This type of rice is the seed of a North American long grain marsh grass, therefore, it is an aquatic grass. Being rich in nutrients and protein, it's easily digestible, which makes it a great option for grain-free vegans who want to fill in nutrition gaps from not eating things like rice and oats. Wheat is the worst of the offenders and should be avoided because it's a highly genetically modified crop and is often grown in poor soil conditions. If you are still having symptoms of inflammation after giving up wheat and gluten, try eliminating soy, corn, and oats since these foods are commonly associated with intolerances. Cardiologist Dr. William Davis, author of *Wheat Belly,* discusses the association between wheat and grains and inflammation in this excerpt from a blog post: Wheat and grains powerfully inflame the body. Inflammation can manifest as facial redness (seborrhea), as other forms of skin rash such as acne, dandruff, eczema, and psoriasis. It can show as joint pain, especially in the hands, wrists, and elbows, sometimes in the knees, hips, and low back. It can show as water retention/edema in the face and ankles. Grain-induced inflammation can also show up as an autoimmune disease: anything from rheumatoid arthritis, to autoimmune pancreatic beta cell destruction (type 1 diabetes), to pernicious anemia (autoimmune destruction of the parietal cells of the stomach responsible for vitamin B12 absorption).[65]

---

65   Dr. William Davis, May 6, 2015, Lose the wheat and grains, lose the inflammation, http://www.wheatbellyblog.com/2015/05/lose-the-wheat-and-grains-lose-the-inflammation/.

If you suffer from any of the above-mentioned health issues, going grain-free may just set you free. The foundation and success of your diet lays in eating large amounts of greens in salads, juices, and smoothies! Replace your grains with greens, nuts, seeds, and sprouts.

Tips for Being a Grain-Free Vegan:

1. Replace grain flour with grain-free flours like coconut or nut flours. You can grind any nut into flour in a high-speed blender or food processor.

2. Soak and sprout nuts and seeds for better digestion and nutrient absorption. You can grow your own sprouts at home or purchase them and add them to salads. Sprouts are the most nutritious plants on the planet.

3. Crowd out other foods by eating primarily fruits and vegetables in large amounts. A dinner salad can consist of large amounts of greens: 1-2 heads of kale or romaine with spinach and plenty of other vegetables included.

4. Clean out your kitchen! Get rid of everything that is processed, gluten filled, preservative laden, and full of sugar. Stock your kitchen and pantry with only the best life-giving foods and those will be the foods you eat! To help your family get on board with your healthier habits, you might consider having a heart to heart conversation about why you want the change. Your influence will set a good example and your loved ones may even follow suit in time. Find peace in knowing that you are doing your whole family a favor by eating in a way that supports life.

Fiber keeps you full, and by filling up with plenty of fruits, vegetables, plant-based protein, and water, being full should not be a problem on a plant-based diet. The key is to keep your fridge stocked and bring enough food with you when you go places. Keep trail mixes on hand, and easy to-go fruits like bananas, apples, and dried fruits. Get dried fruits and trail mixes that are natural and that don't contain sulfates, sulfites, partially hydrogenated oils, or extra added sugars. Lara Bars are good to have on hand, and cut up veggie sticks like carrots, celery, and cucumbers with salsa and guacamole make good snacks. You can make your own kale chips or energy bars at home using whole ingredients. Wash a few apples and wrap them up with plastic wrap and you have easy snacks to munch on while on the go. Grain-free vegan eating is fun and delicious!

Shade 3 - The Junk Food Vegan

Whether you are gluten-free, vegan, paleo or not, there is a wrong and a right way to go vegan. There are plenty of vegan junk foods, like French fries, corn dogs, cookies, doughnuts, cakes, and candies. If you can tolerate vegan junk foods, go ahead and indulge once in a while! Eating vegan is fun! However, if something vegan is processed and full of sugar, fried in oil, and super heavy, it is still a junk food to be avoided. Just because a food is vegan doesn't mean it's good for you or particularly healthy. Simply giving up animal foods does not ensure great health.

Once you shift to a cleaner way of eating, you won't feel so hot after eating the junk. After years of feeling less than great and often with food remorse, I found alternative recipes to satisfy every food craving and indulgence, whether it is rich, creamy, chocolatey, crunchy, salty, or sweet. For example, avocados make foods rich and creamy thus replacing butter. Avocados can be processed with dates to make puddings, frosting, and mousses. Coconut cream can replace dairy cream. Junk food cravings are a thing of the past for me now. Vegan junk foods are great in that they are available for those who are transitioning and can consume them without any adverse reactions. French fries, soy "chicken" nuggets, meat substitutes, ice creams, and cheeses are fun foods, BUT if you are breaking out, gaining weight, or having digestive issues after consuming them, it's best to avoid them.

Shade 4 - Soy-Free Vegan

Soy foods can be problematic and even harmful to your health. This is due to processed, genetically modified soybeans. Whole and organic, fermented soy foods can be beneficial in small amounts. These foods include tempeh, miso, edamame (whole soybeans), tamari (gluten-free soy sauce), and organic tofu. If you have any digestive discomforts or skin breakouts after eating soy products, it is best to leave them out for four to six weeks. Re-introduce them if you feel inclined, and if the symptoms re-occur, then leave them out and re-introduce once again. If the symptoms come back again, leave them out for good. Use your discretion when consuming soy and be aware of how your body reacts. Soy is quite a controversial health food. Studies are stacked up against each other on both sides with opposing information. A significant number of doctors and nutritionists agree that soy is a healthful addition to one's diet. However, let's look at both sides so you can have a better understanding about the differences between healthful and harmful soy products. Then you can decide for yourself if you want to consume soy or not.

For years, we have been reading about the heart healthy benefits of soy, such as being high in protein and fiber while being low in fat and cholesterol. The good news is that soy contains vitamins, minerals, and all essential amino acids, which makes it a nutritious meat and egg substitute. People who consume plant-based protein experience better health simply because they are consuming plant foods and not animal foods. People in Asian countries have been consuming small amounts of tofu for ages and have good health. They eat it in small amounts with a lot of vegetables and fish—not as fake meat, cheese, and dessert replacements. For people suffering from obesity and high cholesterol, replacing cheeseburgers with soy foods like tofu can certainly do the body a service by cutting out the saturated fat and cholesterol. Harvard's School of Public Health says, "Even though soy protein has little direct effect on cholesterol, soy foods are good for the heart and blood vessels because they usually replace less healthful choices, like red meat, and because they deliver plenty of polyunsaturated fat, fiber, vitamins, and minerals, and are low in saturated fat."[66]

Research boasting soy benefits has not been completely comprehensive in proving soy's ability to improve certain diseases. Soy has been coined in studies to lower cholesterol, aid in preventing hormone related cancers, and reduce the likelihood of heart disease.[67] Some studies have examined if soy consumption could help prevent osteoporosis and assist women going through menopause by reducing hot flashes and night sweats, and once again the findings were weak or unsupported with evidence.[68] Other studies found that soy was not so keen at reducing symptoms and preventing disease or cancer.[69] Isoflavones are phytoestrogens derived from soy that strengthen or reduce the effects of estrogen in the body. Isoflavones are also known to block thyroid function and cause endocrine disruption. Despite the benefits known to be associated with soy, the conclusions in studies have been weak or insufficient in providing enough evidence.[70] There was a time when I thought soy was my go to protein source, but I no longer believe that all soy products are healthy, because they're not all created equal, and here's where diet could become confusing. There are studies proving that soy is a health hindrance. It is wise to avoid non-organic soy products in non-fermented processed forms. Ninety percent of non-organic soy is genetically modified and sprayed with carcinogenic herbicides.[71]

66   Harvard. TH., Chan. School of Public Health. (2014). Straight Talk About Soy. Retrieved from https://www.hsph.harvard.edu/nutrition-source/2014/02/12/straight-talk-about-soy/
67   Code of Federal Regulations. Health claims: Soy protein and risk of coronary heart disease. 21CFR101.82. 2001
68   Sirtori, C.R., 2001, Risks and Benefits of Soy Phytoestrogens in Cardiovascular Diseases, Cancer, Climacteric Symptoms and Osteoporosis. Retrieved from https://www.ncbi.nlm.nih.gov/pubmed/11522120?dopt=Abstract
69   Barrett, J. R. (2006). The Science of Soy: What Do We Really Know? Environmental Health Perspectives, 114(6), A352–A358.
70   Harvard. TH., Chan. School of Public Health. (2014). Straight Talk About Soy. Retrieved from https://www.hsph.harvard.edu/nutrition-source/2014/02/12/straight-talk-about-soy/
71   Mercola, Dr. J., (2011). Health Articles. Retrieved from https://articles.mercola.com/sites/articles/archive/2011/12/08/the-dirty-little-secret-hidden-in-much-of-your-health-food.aspx

The dangers of soy don't stop there. Even organically grown soybeans naturally contain anti-nutrients such as saponins, soy toxins, phytates, trypsin inhibitors, lectins, and goitrogens. Anti-nutrients block nutrient absorption of essential minerals.[72] Be wary of ingredients such as soy protein isolate, soy protein concentrate, or textured vegetable protein which are common ingredients in protein powders, breakfast cereals, fake meats, pill supplements, and energy bars. Many of these forms of soy are processed with a neurotoxin solvent called Hexane which is a gasoline byproduct. Basically, it's used as a cheap and easy way to separate the soybean oil from the protein. I don't think you want to eat neurotoxins, do you? Here again shows the importance of choosing organic foods. Organic foods provide a government-regulated, third-party-certified refuge from foods produced and processed with toxins and potentially dangerous chemicals. Federal standards for organic foods are created and enforced by the United States Department of Agriculture, and prohibit the use of synthetic inputs that threaten the environment and/or human health, including hexane.[73] Be aware that toxic chemicals are not banned in products marketed as "natural." Who would of thought food could be this complicated? There's more to ponder here. Protease (aka trypsin inhibitors) block protein absorption and cause swelling of the pancreas, which over time could do serious damage. The pancreas would have to produce more enzymes to digest the food properly, which creates stress and could lead to cancer.[74] Lectins are irritating to the gastrointestinal tract, and high levels of antinutrient oxalates can cause kidney stones.[75] Oxalates have a role in many plant foods in nature to protect them from predators like animals, insects and even humans. Since the oxalates block digestion, the plant seeds can pass through the digestive system, thus spreading and reproducing. Traditional fermentation destroys most of these anti-nutrients, which allows your body to enjoy soy's nutritional benefits in small amounts.

Most Westerners do not consume fermented soy, but rather *unfermented soy,* mostly in the form of soy milk, tofu, textured vegetable protein, and soy infant formula. People who want to feed their children plant-based formulas because they are allergic or think it's healthier often turn to soy-based formulas. I did this with my daughter when she was a baby, and now I am learning about how infant formulas are high in manganese and that high levels of manganese can cause brain damage in infants. My daughter did not turn out brain damaged and she is quite smart, but high levels of manganese have been shown to lower intelligence, and I wish I had known then what I know

72   Munir Cheryan & Joseph J. Rackis (2009) Phytic acid interactions in food systems, C R C Critical Reviews in Food Science and Nutrition, 13:4, 297-335, DOI: 10.1080/10408398009527293
73   The Cornicopia Institute. (2010). Hexane Soy. Retrieved from https://www.cornucopia.org/2010/11/hexane-soy/
74   Kaayla, D.T., (2018) How Soy Wreaks Havoc on Digestion and the Pancreas. Retrieved from https://www.thehealthyhomeeconomist.com/not-just-bad-for-hormones-how-soy-harms-digestion-and-stresses-the-pancreas/
75   Al-Wahsh IA1, Horner HT, Palmer RG, Reddy MB, Massey LK. (2005). Oxalate and Phytate of Soy Foods. Retrieved from https://www.ncbi.nlm.nih.gov/pubmed/15998131

now.[76] Nobody would want to even run that risk of exposure after hearing that. This is a word of caution for people considering feeding their child soy-based formulas.

A great alternative to soy sauce is coconut aminos, which is a soy-free flavor enhancer. Hemp tofu is also available on the market as a soy-free tofu alternative. It is not a good idea to rely on soy products for protein. Many vegan products on the market are made up of soy because it easily replaces the cheese, milk, and meat products most people are accustomed to. You will find soy milk, tofu, soy chorizo, soy ice cream, soy cream cheese, soy cheese, and more as replacements on the shelves. If you can consume soy products with no adverse side effects then make sure they are organic (avoid hexane), but still have small amounts. I have found that I am intolerant to most unfermented soy products, so I avoid them. Many people are discovering intolerances to soy and this is not surprising since many of these products are processed and unnatural.

You want to crowd out processed foods from your diet, even if they are "health" foods, like soy hot dogs or gluten-free vegan pizza. If you are having indigestion, gas, rashes, cramping, constipation, diarrhea, or breakouts after eating soy products then you should avoid them altogether. A majority of animal feed contains soy and is being fed to livestock. If you are consuming the animals, then you are consuming the soy. Even chickens fed soy will lay eggs that contain soy, so if you are consuming the eggs, then you are consuming soy. If you have a strong soy intolerance or allergy, this is useful information for you.

Edamame is the whole food soybean, and when consumed in moderation, it is healthy and nutritious. Finding alternative foods like milks, cheeses, pizzas, and burgers that are soy-free is not difficult either. Companies like Daiya and Kite Hill make excellent vegan, soy-free cheeses and dairy product alternatives like yogurt, cheese, cakes, and pizzas as well. Many veggie burgers can be found soy-free and gluten-free, like Sunshine Burgers, Amy's Sonoma Veggie Burger, Qrunch Foods, Hillary's Eat Well, Dr. Praeger's, Bahama Rice Burgers, and Beyond Meat burger. Let's not forget that the best veggie burgers are the ones you make at home, and they happen to be the most cost effective.

76   Mercola, Dr. J., (2010). Warning: Please Avoid Feeding Manganese to Your Child. Retrieved from https://articles.mercola.com/sites/articles/archive/2010/10/18/manganese-can-adversely-affect-childrens-intelligence.aspx

Shade 5 - Paleo-ish Vegan

In the world of diet and nutrition, the term "paleo" refers to eating as our ancient ancestors did. Essentially, they foraged meat, nuts, berries, vegetables, and tubers. A paleo diet takes out dietary offenders like processed foods, sugar, gluten, and dairy. The paleo diet is touted for balancing hormones, shedding excess weight, reducing inflammation, increasing sex drive, building a stronger immune system, and reducing the risk of cancer from an increased consumption of fruits and vegetables. This sounds incredible, doesn't it?

Well, what if you don't want to eat meat? Can you survive healthfully eating this way? This category of vegan is specific, but effective for increasing beauty, energy, and fat loss. Yes, it can be done in a skillful way. In a sense, you are avoiding grains, dairy products, and legumes, thus sticking to fruits, vegetables, nuts, tubers, and seeds. This sounds a lot like raw-vegan but is less restrictive, and is perfect for those who want to transform their health and beauty but do not want to be eating raw all the time. I don't think it's completely necessary to exclude sprouted foods like lentils or chickpeas if you can tolerate them.

You can include cooked foods like sweet potatoes, squashes, soups, yams, roots, vegetables, and sea vegetables. Protein powders are available now that are paleo friendly, and you can bake foods using coconut and other nut flours to replace grain flours. Eggs can be replaced with chia, ground psyllium husk, or flax seed "eggs," and sugar can be replaced with sweet fruits like dates, applesauce, and bananas. Create this plant-based "egg" binder for recipes by mixing 1 tablespoon of hot water to 3 tablespoons of the seed (flax, chia, or psyllium husk) and let it set a few minutes until it makes a gel. I've spent plenty of nights testing and creating different paleo vegan breads and muffins, and it's easy to find recipe ideas on social media outlets like Pinterest. Baked sweet potato fries with garlic and rosemary used to be a weekly staple for me. You can create delicious soups with ingredients like butternut squash, tomatoes, and fresh herbs. This way of eating is perfect for fall and winter seasons as the weather goes from cooler to cold in most places, and you may desire more warming foods like soups and squashes to balance your system. Fruits are cooling foods, and they work very well in larger amounts for people in the spring and summertime. Some of my favorite fall and winter fruits are persimmons and figs.

For added protein and essential omega fatty acids, I recommend adding hemp seeds and chia seeds to your salads and recipes. These two ingredients are staples in my kitchen. Check out a seasonality chart that corresponds to the area you live in to see what foods are in season and when. Eating foods that are in season are the best foods for you to thrive off of. Local, in-season foods also tend to be more affordable than out-of-season, imported food.

Quinoa is a great gluten-free food to have and is technically a seed. People might be confused and think that quinoa is a grain, but it's considered a pseudo grain. Science tells us that quinoa is a super food since it contains all the essential amino acids, which is rare in plant foods. In addition, quinoa contains nutrients like B vitamins, potassium, antioxidants, calcium, iron, phosphorus, and vitamin E. While quinoa is indeed a wonder food, there is, surprisingly, information out there that might steer one away from eating it. Quinoa contains saponin, which makes a soapy substance when combined with water. Research claims that saponin binds with minerals such as iron, zinc, and calcium, which explains why these saponins cancel out the full nutritional benefits. The British Journal of Nutrition, in its article *The Biological Actions of Saponins in Animal Systems,* states:

> Saponins are steroid or triterpenoid glycosides, common in many plants and plant products that are important in human and animal nutrition. Several biological effects have been ascribed to saponins. Saponins and have also been found to significantly affect growth, feed intake and reproduction in animals and contain anti-nutritional substances such as tannins, phytic acid, and trypsin inhibitors. These structurally diverse compounds have also been observed to kill protozoans and mollusks, impair the digestion of protein and the uptake of vitamins and minerals in the gut, to cause hypoglycemia, and to act as antifungal and antiviral agents.[77]

These compounds can affect animals in a host of different ways both positive and negative. Despite this scientific discussion, I think quinoa is still a healthy gluten and grain-free alternative as a part of a vegan diet. There's a lot worse you could be eating. It seems there is something wrong with everything there is to eat these days, so don't worry. This is more about being informed and making educated choices for yourself.

Beans and legumes can pose a problem as well since they also contain phytic acid and FODMAPS. FODMAPS are short chain carbohydrates and sugar alcohols found in foods naturally or as food additives. They contain a certain carbohydrate called galacto oligosaccharides, which can cause

---

77   The biological action of saponins in animal systems: a review, George Francis1, Zohar Kerem2, Harinder P. S. Makkar3 and Klaus Becker. Department of Aquaculture Systems and Animal Nutrition, Institute for Animal Production in the Tropics and Subtropics, University of Hohenheim (480), D 70593 Stuttgart, Germany, Institute of Biochemistry, Food Science and Nutrition, Faculty of Agricultural, Food and

digestive problems and undesired effects, like gas and bloating. People who suffer from irritable bowel syndrome or other digestive problems are especially affected by FODMAPS.

We must also remember that food is not a religion, and you are not bound to rules and regulations. Remain flexible and in tune to what your current needs are and what your situation calls for and adjust as necessary. Love yourself and make the best choices you can for how you want to look and feel. This is about learning information and finding what works best for you. A vegan beauty can slide day to day between paleo-vegan, raw-vegan, or gluten-free vegan as she sees fit. You have the power to choose what goes in your body and nobody regrets eating beauty foods such as fruits and vegetables. They don't give you the food remorse that French fries, pizza, and ice cream give you. In fact, fruits and veggies make you feel happier, lighter, beautiful, energetic, and vibrant. Who doesn't want to feel that way? You can eat delicious food and desserts without feeling terrible afterwards. It's like having your cake and eating it, too.

Shade 6 - Gluten-Free Vegan

You have decided to try out the vegan diet and you are still experiencing some issues like breakouts, brain fog, mood swings, or poor digestion. You have decided there's no way you are going to give up beans and grains, so at least consider how gluten is impacting your health. Maybe you're thinking you need to go back to eating animal products again because the vegan diet isn't working out for you. That is not necessary. Like finding your correct shade of concealer, you need to find your shade of vegan. It could be something you are eating within the vegan diet that is not agreeing with you, and this is an easy fix. Try avoiding gluten. I never realized how gluten was impacting my health until I cut it out and then had it again. I noticed feeling bloated, foggy-headed, and lethargic after eating it. After giving it up, I felt miles better.

It's quite easy to follow a gluten-free vegan lifestyle, and gluten sensitivities are becoming more and more common because of evolution in crop production. Gluten lurks in white flour, bread products, sauces, processed foods, and meat substitutes like seitan (which is made up of primarily wheat gluten). Gluten is the protein found in grains, and it acts like a glue, keeping everything together while giving foods a soft, chewy texture.

Environmental Quality Sciences, The Hebrew University of Jerusalem, Israel 3Animal Production and Health Section, International Atomic Energy Agency, August 2002.

No matter which kinds of gluten-free foods you eat, if you are gluten intolerant or have celiac disease, you will feel better than if you were eating their gluten counterpart. There is a method to this style of eating that gives the greatest benefit in terms of health and beauty. The method is simply to replace your favorite gluten-filled ingredients with gluten-free alternatives. Stick to whole foods and have the refined gluten-free junk foods in moderation, including gluten-free beer and wine, which, of course, is naturally gluten-free! The gluten-free vegan can eat all plant-based foods except those containing gluten because they have a gluten intolerance, a gluten sensitivity, or they hands-down feel better omitting it from their diet. The method to going gluten-free is easy when you know what contains gluten so you can replace those ingredients with alternatives. Gluten-free grains are rice, sorghum, millet, amaranth, buckwheat, and gluten-free oats. Legumes are gluten-free, like black, kidney, garbanzo, and white beans, as well as red, green, and black lentils. Stock your pantry with gluten-free staples like pasta sauce, tamari (gluten-free soy sauce), and whole beans. Potatoes are gluten-free, as well as many pastas created from gluten-free foods like corn, lentils, quinoa, and brown rice.

The gluten-free industry has been on the rise with product sales that have risen from $11.5 billion to $23 billion. Those sales include products labeled as gluten-free, not including naturally gluten-free foods like produce and meats. Remember that not all gluten-free foods are healthy or budget friendly. Take into consideration that a Glutino Original New York Style Bagel has 26% more calories, 250% more fat, 43% more sodium, 50% less fiber, and double the sugar of Thomas' Plain Bagels.[78] That Glutino bagel is also 74% more expensive than the Thomas' brand, and other products go as far as costing three times as much as their gluten counterpart.

Feeling energized, healthy, and with good digestion are the reasons why the gluten-free vegan should avoid all the processed gluten-free foods and stick to whole foods, like whole grains (excluding wheat, barley, and rye), legumes, fruits, vegetables, nuts, and seeds. You won't feel heavy or bloated. Below is a list of foods and ingredients to avoid when following a gluten-free vegan diet.

- Wheat
- Barley
- MSG Modified Food Starch
- Extenders and Binders
- Maltodextrin (wheat or corn based)
- Hydroxypropylated Starch
- Oil frying could cause cross contamination
- Spelt
- Rye
- Textured/Hydrolyzed Vegetable/ Plant Protein
- Natural Flavors

---

78   fortune.com, We're in a gluten-free bubble that is about to burst, Vikram Mansharamani, May 5, 2015.

- Smoke Flavors
- Dry Roasted Nuts
- Vitamin supplements containing gluten
- Emmer
- Dextrin
- Maltose
- Artificial Flavors
- Natural Colors
- Baking Powder (commonly contains grains - wheat/corn)
- Graham
- Non-Dairy Creamer
- Hydrogenated Starch
- Hydrolysate
- Artificial Colors
- Caramel Color and Flavoring
- Soy Sauce
- Farina
- Farro
- Semolina
- Durum Seasonings (check labels)
- Vegetable Gum
- Vegetable Protein
- Certain Miso Brands
- Bouillon Cubes
- Instant Teas and Coffees

Traditionally, foods like rice, quinoa, oats, amaranth, buckwheat, teff, millet, sorghum, and corn are not labeled as containing gluten, however, they could have effects like gluten. If you are consuming these grains/pseudo grains, try a high raw/paleo-vegan diet. For some people, having gluten in small amounts may trigger a reaction. Get to know your triggers.

Shade 7 - Raw Vegan/ High Raw Vegan

The purest style of vegan is what's been around ever since the beginning of time, and that is the raw vegan diet. We started out on earth with only fruits, vegetables, nuts, and seeds, and over time, humanity has evolved to cook and process foods. Raw vegan is my favorite! To preserve the enzymes and full nutritional value of foods, nothing is heated above 118°F. This style of eating is great for those who have a strong desire to engage in it, or who have serious health and beauty goals. It will revolutionize your life in the most epic way imaginable. Sustaining oneself on this diet does require a bit of planning and learning about how to find easy recipes you love, as well as how to make it affordable for you. Eating only raw fruits and vegetables, nuts and seeds is a luxury, and our food system is structured in such a way that keeps the cost of organic produce quite high. Here are some tips for keeping a raw vegan diet affordable.

1. Buy in bulk. Stores like Costco carry a lot of organic produce at a fraction of the cost. Also, grocery stores often discount produce ordered by the case. Just ask the produce manager about ordering this way for deals.

2. Shop the farmer's markets. I have seen persimmons sold for $2.99 each in grocery stores and $2.00/lb at the farmer's market. If you go to the market right as its closing, vendors will usually give discounts to sell what is left for the day, making it the perfect time to ask for deals.

3. Buy in-season and locally.

To stay healthy on a raw vegan diet, it's important to eat a balance of fruits, fats, and greens. Greens balance fruit and their sugars. If you eat too many fats or fruit without the addition of greens, you can run into problems, such as feeling spacy, heavy, ungrounded, and lacking in vital minerals that greens provide. As a high raw vegan, 80-90% of your diet should consist of raw foods and 10-20% of cooked foods. Let's say you're loving raw foods, but you still want to eat hot soup, baked squash, beans, or quinoa from time to time. Great! I find this style highly sustainable for the dedicated vegan who would like to reap all the benefits of raw foods without feeling restricted. Unless you have a strong conviction about eating 100% raw, there is no reason to deprive yourself of life-sustaining whole foods that were created by nature.

The raw vegan lifestyle is cleansing in and of itself; you may wish to maintain it for a set amount of time to accomplish health goals for cleansing purposes, or to jumpstart a healthier lifestyle. The body is constantly renewing cells and excreting waste. Each day and month, your body is regenerating itself and organ cells are being renewed. The only parts not believed to renew are heart cells and brain neurons. Liver cells are known to renew every 300-500 days, gut lining cells last about half a week, and your skin renews itself every 2-4 weeks. This is fascinating because we can improve the health of our cells based on the high quality nutrition we choose to build them with. Therefore, we are not stuck with the same sick cells if they are regenerating constantly. Healing can occur with raw fruits and vegetables and their juices. People run into problems when the systems become intoxicated and blocked after years of stress, a lack of exercise, and improper nutrition. The body is unable to take out the trash and disease can occur. Instead, adopt a lifestyle that facilitates healing, prevents disease, premature aging, and gives life.

Supplementation

No matter the route to veganism you prefer, or whether you slide back and forth between all of them, a bit of supplementation is necessary to ensure your body is getting what it needs. Vitamin B-12 is an essential nutrient found mostly in animal products but can also be found in nutritional yeast, tofu, and seaweeds. We generally do not eat enough of those foods to fulfill the B-12 requirements for our bodies. At the very least, make sure you take a vitamin B-12 supplement. I recommend taking a quality multivitamin/multimineral supplement sourced from food, not chemicals.

Not all supplements are created equal because some use chemical vitamin ingredients. It's important to get vitamins sourced from foods so they can be recognized and absorbed into the body. Vitamin D is another important nutrient that 70% of the U.S population is deficient in.[79] Dr. Weil recommends that everyone takes a daily supplement of 2,000 IU D3. Vitamin D is found in mushrooms, especially shiitake mushrooms. Your body can make its own vitamin D by simply being exposed to the sun. Isn't that fascinating? Make sure to expose your body to the sun as much as possible, or for at least 15-20 minutes a day. During the winter, this is more difficult since sunshine may be limited. Many people become depressed during the times of year when exposure to sunlight is limited. The phenomenon is called seasonal affective disorder and light therapy can be effective for up to 80% of sufferers. Light boxes can be purchased, and they give out a full spectrum of light like that of the sun.

It's best to eat your vitamins as food rather than as supplements because that is the best way for your body to get what it needs. Eating quality plant-based fat in moderate amounts is important for vegans and can be found in delicious foods such as nut butters, nuts, coconuts, coconut oil, olives, avocados, flax oil, and olive oil. The human body does not need as much protein as you might imagine, and you can get more than enough to meet your protein requirements eating anywhere from an original vegan diet to a raw vegan diet. Protein is a macronutrient that is commonly over consumed. High protein, high fat diets have become popular due to their short-term weight loss effects. When carbohydrate energy stores are depleted, the body turns to fat for energy use. High protein diets produce weight loss due to a reduction of calorie consumption, not an increase in protein, and are not sustainable.

Unfortunately, these diets are low in fiber and can cause long term health problems. High protein diets are associated with osteoporosis, cancer, cardiovascular disease, impaired kidney func-

79   Light Therapy, Dr. Weil, drweil.com

tion, and weight loss issues.[80] A report by the Physicians Committee for Responsible Medicine ana-lyzed 429 people following a high protein, low carbohydrate, high fat diet through an online registry in 2004. The largest percentage of participants reported constipation, loss of energy, and bad breath. More complications reported included difficulty concentrating, kidney problems, heart problems, and more.[81]

Carbohydrates are an important macro nutrient in addition to protein, and they play a critical role in protein absorption. Eating whole grains, nuts, and seeds from plant-based sources increases protein absorption because the carbohydrates release insulin. The insulin helps your muscles absorb amino acids, especially before and after exercise. A plant-based diet rich in fruits, vegetables, legumes, and whole grains is sustainable long-term and helps keep the weight off. Research by T. Colin Campbell in his widely acclaimed book *The China Study* has proven that consuming more than 10% protein from animal sources turns on cancer markers in cells, and the higher the percentage of animal protein consumed, the higher the percentage of cancer cell receptors activate. Campbell was also able to conclude that plant-based protein did not turn on cancer cells at all, which makes a strong case for avoiding animal products at large.[82]

It's fascinating that 100 calories of ground beef yields 10 grams of protein, while 100 calories of spinach yields around 12 grams. You would have to eat nearly 15 cups or a 16 oz package of spinach to reach 100 calories! Yes, that's a lot of spinach, but the point is you can get enough protein from eating fruits and vegetables. Meat and animal products are not necessary for you to meet your daily nutritional requirements. This protein chart lays out the amounts of protein contained in common plant foods.

80   http://www.pcrm.org/health/diets/vegdiets/how-can-i-get-enough-protein-the-protein-myth
81   Physicians Committe for Responsible Medicine. 2004. Analysis of Health Problems Associated with High-Protein, High-Fat, Carbohy-drate-Restricted Diets. Retrieved from http://www.pcrm.org/health/reports/analysis-of-health-problems-associated-with-high
82   Campbell, T.C., & Campbell, T.M. II., (2006). The China Study. Dallas, TX, Benbella Books

Protein Percentage Chart[83]

Vegetables %		Vegetables %		Grains %		Fruits %		Nuts & Seeds %	
Spinach	49	Artichokes	22	Wild Rice	16	Lemon	16	Pumpkin Seeds	21
Watercress	46	Cabbage	22	Buckwheat	15	Honeydew Melon	10	Sunflower Seeds	17
Kale	45	Celery	21	Oatmeal	15	Cantaloupe	9	Walnuts	13
Broccoli	45	Eggplant	21	Millet	12	Strawberry	8	Sesame Seeds	13
Brussel Sprouts	44	Tomatoes	18	Brown Rice	8	Orange	8	Almonds	12
Turnip Greens	43	Onions	16	Amaranth	13	Blackberry	8	Cashews	12
Collards	43	Beets	15			Cherry	8	Brazil Nuts	8
Cauliflower	40	Pumpkin	12			Apricot	8	Pecans	5
Mustard Greens	39	Potatoes	11			Grape	8	Quinoa	15
Mushrooms	38	Yams	8			Watermelon	8		
Chinese Cabbage	34	Sweet Potatoes	6			Tangerine	7		
Parsley	34	Sunflower Sprouts	25			Papaya	6		
Lettuce	34	Sprouts	25-35			Peach	6		
Green Peas	30	Lentils	29			Pear	5		
Zucchini	28	Garbanzo Beans	23			Banana	5		
Green Beans	26	Mung Bean Sprouts	43			Grapefruit	5		
Cucumbers	24	Spirulina	65-70			Pineapple	3		
Dandelion Greens	24	Black Beans	15 grams/1 cup			Apple	1		
Green Pepper	22	Tempeh	31 grams/1 cup						

83   Nutritive Value of American Foods, USDA Agriculture Handbook No. 456, Paul C. Bragg, Miracle of Fasting, pg. 233.

Iron is an important dietary micronutrient that can be obtained from plants. Iron absorption is increased by consuming vitamin C and iron foods together.

Plant Based Iron Sources[84]

Food	Amount	Iron (mg)
Soybeans	1 cup	8.8
Blackstrap Molasses	2 Tbsp	7.2
Lentils	1 cup	6.6
Spinach	1 cup	6.4
Chickpeas – cooked	1 cup	4.7
Tempeh	1 cup	4.5
Swiss Chard	1 cup	4.0
Kidney Beans	1 cup	3.9
Black Beans	1 cup	3.6
Pinto Beans	1 cup	3.6
Quinoa – cooked	1 cup	8
Tahini	2 Tbsp	2.7
Peas – cooked	1 cup	2.5
Cashews	¼ cup	2.1
Bok Choy – cooked	1 cup	1.8
Raisins	½ cup	1.6
Apricots – dried	15 halves	1.4
Watermelon	⅛ medium	1.4
Almonds	¼ cup	1.3
Kale	1 cup	1.2
Sunflower Seeds	¼ cup	1.2
Broccoli	1 cup	1.1
Tomato Juice	8 ounces	1.0
Sesame Seeds	2 Tbsp	1.0
Brussel Sprouts	1 cup	.9

84 USDA Branded Food Products Database, ndb.nal.usda.gov, 6/18/2015

CHAPTER 10

TIME TO GET RAW

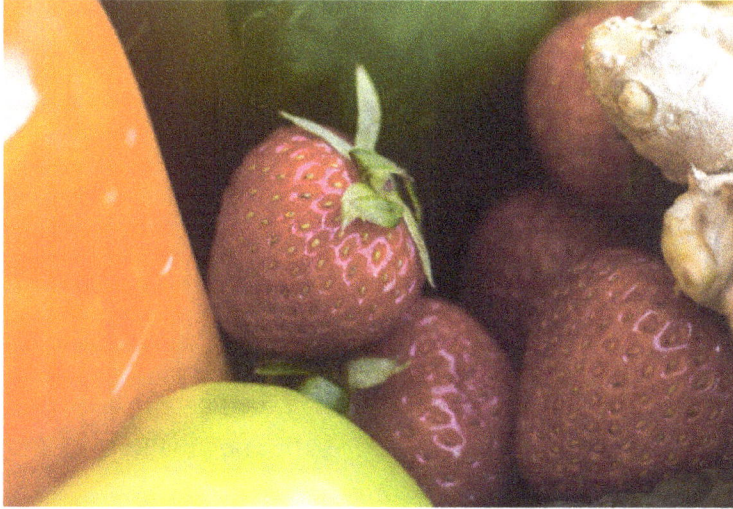

Raw foods are life-giving, and they also love you back in so many ways. This is why I love eating raw fruits and vegetables. Don't judge! Raw vegans don't just chew on carrots and lettuce all day long, and the benefits of eating raw foods benefit the body, mind, and spirit.

Starting with the body, raw foods energize and prevent disease. If you were to bury a raw apple in some soil, it would decompose into the earth and seeds would sprout, growing new life. If you were to bake that same apple and then plant it in the ground, it would not grow because it is already dead. Putting cooked food in our bodies may nourish us, but it does not give the same kind of life, regeneration, and healing that raw foods give. Eating raw also keeps you slim, youthful, energized, more balanced, and reverses aging. This is very powerful. Filling your body with quality nutrition, antioxidants, and enzymes keeps the cells alive and regenerated. You will see notable improvements in the way you look and feel.

Why should you eat primarily raw? By not heating your food above 115-118°F, nutrition is enhanced. Cooking decreases nutritional value and enzymes in food. When food is raw or heated only up to104-118°F, the enzymes and life are preserved in order to nourish, restore, rejuvenate, and slow down aging. The raw food energy is then used by the body to energize, give life to your cells, fight disease, pain, and even cancer. Cooked plant-based foods are still healthy and nourishing, however. It is up to you how much of both raw and cooked foods you want to incorporate into your diet based on your needs and the results you want. You will notice a difference in how you feel eating cooked foods after eating more raw foods or 100% raw for a period of time.

Some people argue that certain foods are better for you when cooked. Some claim that tomatoes and broccoli, for example, are more nutritious and digestible when cooked. Eating 100% raw is not for everybody, however, you might go 50/50 or 80/20. It doesn't have to be all or nothing. You could eat raw until dinner time and then include cooked vegetables with your evening meal. It is a personal choice and can be used for periods of time for desired results or for cleansing and rejuve-nation.

I find raw food easy to digest, especially if taken with digestive enzymes, and I used to have the worst digestion. I like to run broccoli and cauliflower through the food processor to rice it. It can then easily be added to salads with your favorite dressings or blended with other veggies and spices to make pâtés or burgers for wraps or lettuce leaf filling. This is an easy way to consume raw broccoli and cauliflower.

People often toil over bread and have this love-hate relationship with it. I say, *Who needs bread?* Try replacing bread with collard and romaine leaves by making homemade wraps. Collard and romaine leaves are easy to use, much more nutritious than most breads and crackers, and are beauty giving! My broccoli sundried tomato pâté in the recipe section is an easy and delicious way to eat raw cauliflower and broccoli.

Another benefit of a raw vegan diet is great elimination due to the high fiber and water content of the foods. Eating fruits with greens and fats, such as romaine lettuce and avocado, creates a balance, helps stabilize blood sugar, and prolongs energy levels. Fruit is the best beauty and energy food, and it keeps your body hydrated and beaming. Fruit meals are ideal for athletes, fitness addicts, working moms, or pretty much anybody who needs a lot of energy and does not have a lot of time to waste being tired. Isn't this everybody? We live in such a fast paced, busy world. Fruit is true fast food! You do not have to worry about counting calories and carbs when you are eating raw/vegan meals, mono-fruit meals, and following simple food combining principles. Who wants to count calories, measure, and weigh food? You have more important things to focus on in life, like the things bringing you joy and the people you love.

Purchasing a juicer and making fresh juice at home is a great way to increase energy, beauty, and reel back the years for anti-aging. Yes! You can get better with age. People who live a raw food lifestyle look up to ten years younger than they are. This has been my experience, since people tell me I look younger than my actual age. People spend thousands of dollars on medical procedures to look younger, but by consuming fresh juice and smoothies, you are drinking from the fountain of youth. The power of raw fruits and vegetables ease the wrinkles from your face and bring about an inner glow that cannot be purchased from a bottle. Even more powerfully necessary than the beauty component to all of this is the heightened clarity of consciousness and increased feelings of happiness that eating raw beauty foods can bring.

Food affects the psyche, meaning it affects our mood, productivity, relationships, and our ability to contribute to the world in a positive way. Food has energy in it, and by that, I mean the life or lack of it is transferred into our being. If we eat chemicals, processed sugar, and meat from animals who lived lives of pain, suffering and fear, the energy we receive from that food is not going to be as great as the energy we receive from raw fruits and vegetables, which transfer high vibrations of energy and life from the sun into your body when you eat them. Cooked food does not have the same effect. Raw plants induce natural feelings of peace and a positive disposition,[85] whereas refined sugar and carbohydrates, combined with caffeine and alcohol tend to induce aggressive feelings.[86] People who eat more raw fruits and vegetables will feel and age better than those who don't. Annette Larkins is in her mid-seventies and has been vegetarian for over 54 years. She's been raw vegan for around 30 years, has incredible energy and looks ridiculously amazing on top of that. Another raw vegan beauty is Karyn Calabrese who is 71 and has been eating raw for over 30 years. Part of what makes her so inspiring is she takes professional ballet classes with 22-year olds, has done yoga for 30 years and helps chronically sick people get well with the power of detoxing/raw foods.[87] Great health consists of a happy, positive mind, with plenty of energy to get through the day, good digestion, elimination, sound relationships, physical activity, and gratitude for the blessings given to us in life. Clearly, there is more contributing to health than food, but food is the foundation for which all else is built upon.

85   Renaissance Humans Blog Post, (2018), Why You Feel Happier on a Raw Food Diet. Retrieved from http://renaissancehumans.com/why-people-feel-better-on-raw-food-diets/
86   Deans, E., MD., (March 1, 2012). Do Carbs Make You Crazy? Evidence that blood glucose and dietary carbohydrate affect mood. Retrieved from https://www.psychologytoday.com/us/blog/evolutionary-psychiatry/201203/do-carbs-make-you-crazy
87   The Fruit Doctor. (2018) The Karyn Effect: 65-year-old raw vegan. Retrieved from http://www.thefruitdoctor.com/the-karyn-effect-karyn-calabrese-65-year-old-raw-vegan/

When you eat in a way that promotes cleansing on an ongoing basis via a raw food or high raw diet, it feels as if the aging process reverses and slows down. I look better now than I did ten and twenty years ago. I credit this to my high raw diet! People who start eating raw often transform and look years younger as a result. You can regain your vitality, look ravishing, improve your self-image, and slim down with raw foods.

Many popular food items like tacos, pizza, and cookies can be recreated just like your favorites in ways that support your health and beauty goals. Try fruits and vegetables you have never tried before as there are so many varieties. Have you ever had fresh young coconut, jackfruit, or cherimoyas? They are delicious! I am excited for you to try new foods you will love. For those who want to incorporate more raw foods into their diet, a good way to start is to replace one meal and snacks with raw foods. This method works well for many people, is simple, and I like to call it the high-raw diet. Here is a food pyramid displaying the hierarchy of foods to consume on a raw food diet. The majority is obviously water and greens, moving up to fruits and vegetables, with small amounts of nuts, seeds, herbs, and fats.

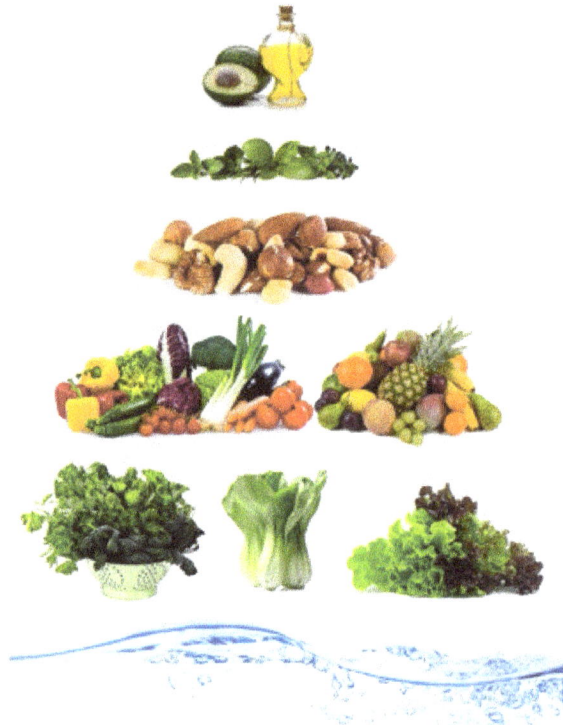

Not only will your cells be fueled, regenerated, and energized, but your mind will be renewed. Eating raw foods feels like magic because energy is released into your being, causing your mind and body to be transformed with clarity. You might even crave exercise, and experience a sense of calm, spiritual connectedness springing forward. Many people attest to the power raw foods have given them to revolutionize their life. Serena Williams, the famous tennis player, was so sick with an autoimmune condition known as Sjogren's syndrome that it nearly ended her career. She used the raw vegan diet to regain her health, which allowed her to continue playing tennis. You can also use this lifestyle as I have to overcome health challenges and regain your health in ways you have never thought possible.

Another benefit of raw foods is glowing beauty from within. All too often, women are focused on what products to put on their skin or what procedures can be done to look younger and more beautiful. When the body is cleansed with raw foods, nourished with fruits and vegetables, hydrated with enough water, and well rested, those beauty results are far better and more affordable than relying on potions, lotions, and procedures. I challenge you to go raw for a week to thirty days to see results for yourself. Eating a high raw diet (80-100%) is possible, and people are thriving off this lifestyle.

I'd like to share some science behind this concept. Cooking foods produces advanced glycoxidation which occurs as a result of the cooking process. Dietary advanced glycation end products (dAGES) are known to contribute to increased oxidant stress and inflammation, which are linked to recent epidemics of diabetes and cardiovascular disease.[88] In high amounts, these end products are pathogenic and absorbed by the body. This can increase chronic inflammation, contribute to heart disease, diabetes, aging, hyperglycemia, and cellular damage. Animal products high in fat, fried foods, and barbecued meats are the highest in AGEs, while fruits, vegetables, legumes, and whole grains are lower. Dietary AGEs have also been found to be associated with dysfunction in ovaries in polycystic ovarian syndrome as well as insulin resistance.

Insulin resistance is associated with oxidative stress and inflammation. Significantly reducing AGEs in the diet has favorable effects on hormonal function, ovulation, and metabolic processes.[89] By steaming, boiling, poaching, stewing, or basically cooking with lower temperatures, you decrease the amount of dietary AGE formation in food. Frying, grilling, and roasting yields higher amounts. The

88   Jaime Uribarri, MD, Sandra Woodruff, RD…& Helen Vlassara, MD, Advanced Glycation End Products in Foods and a Practical Guide to Their Reduction in the Diet, Journal of the American Dietetic Association, ncbi.nlm.nih.gov.
89   Garg, Deepika, Merhi, Zaher, Nutrients. 2015 Dec; 7, Advanced Glycation End Products: Link Between Diet and Ovulatory Dysfunction in PCOS? ncbi.nlm.nih.gov

National Cancer Institute found there is one main group of cancer causing chemicals to be concerned with. Those chemicals are called polycyclic aromatic hydrocarbons and they are produced when food (particularly meat) is cooked at high temperatures like pan frying and grilling over an open flame.[90] This information is astounding. Polycyclic aromatic hydrocarbons are also found in car exhaust fumes, smoked foods, and cigarettes, which have been known to cause cancer for decades. Both processed meats and cigarettes are considered category 1 carcinogens. There has been a large movement away from smoking cigarettes, but not away from eating barbecued or smoked foods. Occasional smoked and chargrilled foods are probably okay, but excessive amounts are not. Americans grill food over gas and charcoal all the time. Gas grills only reduce the cancer risk by a small amount, so avoiding these foods is something to take into consideration.[91]

Victoria Boutenko, in her book *12 Steps to Raw Foods*, explains there is ample evidence from basic research of compounds in cooked and processed meats and fish that heterocyclic amines (HCAs) and polycyclic aromatic hydrocarbons (PAHs) are mutated and carcinogenic. Basically, when heating starch-rich foods to high temperatures, a cancer-causing compound called acrylamide is formed and is found in many foods such as chips, French fries, baked potatoes, breakfast cereals, and bread. There has been increased evidence that AGEs might be implicated in the development of chronic degenerative diseases of aging, such as cardiovascular disease, Alzheimer's disease, and with complications of diabetes mellitus.[92] Results of several studies in animal models and humans show that the restriction of dietary AGEs has positive effects on wound healing, insulin resistance, and cardiovascular diseases.[93] According the World Health Organization, processed meats like ham, hot dogs, sausage, bacon, and some lunch meats increases your chances of developing colon cancer.[94] The way food is prepared is important to take into consideration. Raw foods are the best because they reverse disease, increase longevity, and rejuvenate on a cellular level.

The decision to eat meat, fish, and dairy products is personal, and going vegan is a decision a person makes who is interested and willing. There are many pros to adopting a plant-based lifestyle. Eating a plant-based diet does not have to be an all or nothing decision. Some people eat mostly veg-

90   National Cancer Institute. (2017). Chemicals in Meat Cooked at High Temperatures and Cancer Risk. Retrieved from https://www.cancer.gov/about-cancer/causes-prevention/risk/diet/cooked-meats-fact-sheet
91   Looking at Causes of Cancer that you can Avoid, nutritioninstitute.com
92   Takeuchi M1, Kikuchi S, Sasaki N, Suzuki T, Watai T, Iwaki M, Bucala R, Yamagishi S. (2004). [Abstract]. U.S. National Library of Medicine National Institutes of Health. Involvement of advanced glycation end-products (AGEs) in Alzheimer's disease. Retrieved from https://www.ncbi.nlm.nih.gov/pubmed/15975084
93   Luevano-Contreras C, Chapman-Novakofski K, Dietary advanced glycation end products and aging, Pubmed.gov, 2010 Dec;2(12):1247-65.
94   Simon, S., (2015) World Health Organization Says Processed Meat Causes Cancer. Retrieved from https://www.cancer.org/latest-news/world-health-organization-says-processed-meat-causes-cancer.html

an, transitioning over time, whereas others go cold turkey overnight. Going raw is a rewarding way to effortlessly lose weight, have more energy, and look younger. Eating as many raw foods as possible, coupled with stress reduction and exercise, are powerful secrets to looking beautiful. It is worth experimenting with to take your health and beauty to the next level. Be sure to eat enough food so that you are full and taking in enough calories. Chronometer is a great app that allows you to input the food you eat during the day, track micro and macro nutrients and caloric amounts you are consuming. Do this if you are curious, or for a little while to get a feel for how much food you need in a day for your new style of eating. I stopped measuring food, counting calories, and weighing myself years ago. Instead, I listen to my body to direct me on when and what to eat. This takes time and practice, but it's liberating to eat when you're hungry and stop when you're full, free from the duty of food polling.

Therapeutic Benefits of Juicing

Juicing fruits and vegetables is one of the best methods for increasing your energy levels, enhancing your beauty, delivering nutrition, and kicking up the anti-aging process into high gear. Juice therapy is like medicine. It's preventative and life giving. Juice fasting is an age-old remedy for almost anything as it removes the need for digestion while still providing nutrition to the cells. When fasting is practiced, many issues are resolved as the body goes to work on healing itself internally. Smoothies and juices are great ways to nourish the body while creating minimal impact on the digestive system. The whole digestive system gets a break.

Juice fasting, or juice cleansing, is a practical way to fast in modern life, and amazing results can be accomplished through a juice cleanse. The body is still nourished with enzymes, vitamins, and minerals from the juice. This makes it possible to carry on with everyday life and exercise at your discretion. Productivity is increased because you save time you would normally spend preparing and eating food. Juicing allows you to gain mental clarity from carbohydrates and fuel the brain.

Look at some of the age-old benefits of fasting. It gives the body a physiological rest, increases eating pleasure, retrains the taste buds, teaches the body how much food it needs, rejuvenates the system, aids in the elimination process, and energizes the body. This type of fasting allows the body to heal itself as nature's cure. In addition, juicing normalizes cholesterol and blood pressure levels. It can relieve tension, insomnia, aid in detoxification, leading to a more vigorous sex life, and is the fastest way to lose weight.[95] People with blood sugar imbalances should consult a medical doctor before fasting. Fasting can be done once a week for one day, or once monthly, anywhere from one to three days. Fasting a few times a year can be beneficial. Practicing a longer cleanse is great as well to keep the body and mind performing at their best. It's wise to do this with help and/or supervision. While on a fast, you might experience a healing crisis, which might feel bring about fatigue, headaches, depression, or skin rashes. These side effects are temporary since toxins are moving out from your cells.

The best among these beauty elixirs is the famous green juice. Beet, carrot, and citrus juices are wonderful as well. Having a large green juice for breakfast is energizing and can ward off the need for coffee. This means glowing skin and fewer wrinkles for you. Regardless of whether you are supplementing your diet with fresh fruit and vegetable juices or are embarking on a juice cleanse, you will reap the benefits that juices deliver.

Some opinions voice that juice is high in sugar and can lead to weight gain. This is not true. There is a huge difference between what comes out of kale, beets, ginger, lemon, and a Mountain Dew. Yes, carrots and watermelon are higher in sugar, but not the kind of white processed sugar that leads to inflammation and diabetes. Carrot juice is loaded with vitamin A and potassium, which makes it perfect for clearing up skin problems while clearing out toxins in the body by helping the liver do its job. Carrot juice is also great for restoring eyesight and even for helping with inflammatory disease. Tart cherry juice is helpful for adults with chronic insomnia because it contains melatonin, a sleep inducing hormone. A small study shows that by drinking one cup of tart cherry juice twice daily for two weeks, some relief was experienced.[96] It appears the cherry juice helped people sleep better.

Whole food and smoothie cleanses are also an option for people who cannot or do not want to juice fast. Great results can be obtained from smoothies as well. Smoothies are a good option for people who are concerned with blood sugar levels since they contain fiber. Fiber slows the release of sugar into the bloodstream. If you are concerned about the sugar content in freshly made juice, simply blend it with greens like spinach, or other additions like chia seeds, flax seeds, avocado, or coconut oil. These add good fats to the juice and give you longer sustained energy. Chia seeds and flax also add fiber and healthy omega fatty acids that slow down sugar absorption in the bloodstream and add a glow to your skin and hair. Blending spinach into fruit juices can add fiber and iron into the mix also. Iron is more readily absorbed when combined with vitamin C, which makes orange juice blended with spinach and basil a delicious juice combination that will leave you feeling beautiful and energetic any time of day.

95   Paul C. Bragg, Patricia Bragg, N.D., Ph.D; The Miracle of Fasting
96   Liu AG, Tipton RC, Pan W, Finley JW, Prudente A, Karki N, Losso JN, Greenway FL. Tart Cherry Juice Increases Sleep Time in Older Adults with Insomnia. Experimental Biology 2014. San Diego, CA. April 28, 2014.

There is a difference between fresh pressed juices and those that sit on the shelf for days and months. Juices are best consumed right after they are made to get the most nutrition and enzymes available. Be aware of the drinks companies call juices that really aren't juices at all, but merely artificial flavors and sugars mixed with water. Juice bars are popular and are popping up all over the globe. While buying premade juice and visiting juice bars are both easy and convenient, the price adds up quickly. It's a great investment to purchase a juicer to make your own juices at home. Juicers vary in cost and quality. I started out with an affordable model and eventually upgraded to the Omega Vert 350. You can tell if a juicer is of high quality if the pulp it spits out is dry. This means all the water, vitamins, and minerals have been extracted. The pulp can be used in other recipes like veggie burgers, crackers, or as garden compost. You do not have to waste the vegetable matter.

Here is an interesting finding for those interested in athletic performance. A study was done at the University of Exerter's School of Sports and Health Sciences to see how beet juice would affect cycling performance. Because beet juice contains a high number of nitrates, it was found to significantly improve the performance of cyclists who consumed it as opposed to the control group who did not. In fact, the group who drank the beet juice was able to pedal 16% longer with lower resting blood pressure as well.[97] You may want to "just beet it," like Michael Jackson and juice some beets for enhanced athletic performance.

Apples are another fabulous fruit with many different varieties to choose from. Green apples are lower in sugar, which makes them a great choice to use in recipes or juices for those who want to control sugar consumption. Apple juice contains pectin, a water soluble, gel-like substance found in fruits and vegetables. Pectin scrubs out your colon and has a stark laxative effect, helping people with problems going to the bathroom. Constipation is a problem for many people and can rob you of precious energy, beauty, and health. Who is not miserable when they are constipated? Combine fresh apple juice with spinach juice in a 1:1 ratio, throw in some parsley, and you will be better before you know it! Having this juice daily on an empty stomach for a short amount of time is bound to clear any issues around constipation. Spinach not only fights wrinkles naturally, but it also contains minerals and oxalic acid which combine to make a powerful scrubbing inside the colon, thus removing old waste matter that is caked up inside.

An unhealthy colon can cause fatigue, skin problems, impaired mental functioning, pain and stiffness in the joints, bad breath, poor nutrient absorption, irritable bowel syndrome, and more.

97   University of Exeter. "Beetroot Juice Boosts Stamina, New Study Shows." ScienceDaily. ScienceDaily, 7 August 2009. www.sciencedaily.com/releases/2009/08/090806141520.htm

Disease can begin in the colon, and it is wise to try out juicing for yourself to experience the profound effects colon cleansing has on your health. Consume raw fruits, vegetables, and their juices daily to promote natural cleansing and colon health maintenance. There is a time and place for enemas and colonics to assist in deeper colon cleansing as well. They are not something to become dependent on. Have faith in the fiber of fruits and vegetables. Constipation will be a thing of the past once your diet is comprised mostly of these foods.

The difference between smoothies and juices is something commonly confused. Smoothies can be a combination of different whole fruits, juices, superfoods, protein powder, liquids, and/or whole vegetables. They offer a high amount of nutrition and energy in an easily digestible form. Smoothies are full of hydration, vitamins, minerals, enzymes, and fiber. They are fantastic meal replacements and/or pre/post workout snacks. If you want more of a meal smoothie, drink them in larger quantities, whereas if you want a snack, have a smaller amount. Juices offer many of the same benefits as smoothies. The difference is that a juicer will separate the juice from the pulp, thus juices do not contain fiber. Even when consumed with food, fresh fruit and vegetable juices will make you glow from the inside out. It comes down to your preference. Mostly I prefer fresh juices in the morning and a protein smoothie later in the afternoon, before a workout.

Supplements & Adaptogens

Supplements and adaptogens are fun to try and, in some cases, necessary for reaching your highest potential. Other recommendations include vitamin D3, multivitamin/multimineral, omega fatty acids, DHA, and/or others depending on your needs. Some of my favorite supplements to take are herbal adaptogens. Rather than treating symptoms one by one, adaptogenic herbs rebalance the system and help us cope with stress naturally. Rather than increasing or decreasing a specific function in the body, they have been used for thousands of years to balance the body by combating the effects of stress, fatigue, and illness. They even lower cortisol, and I love them!

Adaptogenic herbs were found by Russian scientists to adapt and survive in harsh conditions and, in turn, help people to do the same. Stress affects nearly everybody in different ways, and when stress hits me, I have trained myself to recognize the symptoms and combat them as necessary.

When I am feeling fatigued and anxious, I know it's time to take a step back, meditate, rest, get a massage, pray, journal, and practice saying no to things that are not serving me at the time. That always helps! Stress can induce anxiety, depression, food cravings, binge eating, headaches, indigestion, colds, flus, muscle tension, and more.

Among the most popular adaptogens to help with stress are ginseng, rhodiola, holy basil, ashwagandha, maca, and astragalus root. Maca is something I regularly keep stocked in my kitchen. It's grown in the Peruvian Andes and was used as food and medicine in South America for centuries. Normally purchased as a powder, it's amazing for increased energy, hormonal balance, strength, endurance, fertility, increased libido, blood pressure levels, and relief from depression. Maca can be used in powder form as an energy boost to your daily smoothies. Ginseng, also known as eleuthero (Siberian ginseng), increases stamina and athletic performance, improves blood sugar levels (in type 2 diabetes), protects against cancer, and decreases the chance of catching colds. In addition, the American variety of ginseng is known to improve memory, whereas the Asian variety is known to improve pre/post-menopausal symptoms in women and relieve chronic fatigue syndrome.

Rhodiola is fantastic as a mood enhancer and improves mental and physical performance. This wondrous herb increases energy, endurance, and reduces anxiety. Studies have shown that rhodiola was able to relieve mild to moderate symptoms of depression,[98] and provide significant improvement for people with generalized anxiety disorder.[99] Rhodiola is also used to help cope with stress, increase stamina, energy, and mental function. I personally use rhodiola to help me combat fatigue and to increase my overall feeling of wellbeing. This is one of my favorite herbs because it makes me feel more energetic, uplifted, and stress resistant.

Holy basil or tulsi is among the list of super herbs to sing praises for its ability to protect against environmental stress stemming from toxins. Tulsi also helps to normalize blood sugar levels, blood-fat levels, blood pressure, and boosts cognitive function and memory. Because it is also antimicrobial, it can protect against infection.

Ashwagandha is another super herb that boasts anti-inflammatory, antioxidant, immune balancing, anti-tumor, and anti-anxiety properties. Not only does it calm the central nervous system, but it can relieve arthritis by reducing inflammation. In studies, Ashwagandha was found to suppress

98   Darbinyan V1, Aslanyan G, Amroyan E, Gabrielyan E, Malmström C, Panossian A., (2007) Clinical trial of Rhodiola rosea L. extract SHR-5 in the treatment of mild to moderate depression. Retrieved from https://www.ncbi.nlm.nih.gov/pubmed/17990195
99   Bystritsky A1, Kerwin L, Feusner JD. (2008) A pilot study of Rhodiola rosea (Rhodax) for generalized anxiety disorder (GAD). Retrieved from https://www.ncbi.nlm.nih.gov/pubmed/18307390

the growth of cancer cells related to the breast, prostate, leukemia, and colon.[100] Other noted benefits from taking Ashwagandha include healthier arteries, less stress related tendencies, more muscle strength, improved sexual function, improved memory, and increased endurance.

Cordyceps, chaga, Lion's Mane, and reishi mushrooms are great for energizing the body and keeping the mind alert and focused. Cordyceps and reishi are in the medicinal mushroom family and are a few fungi goodies to take note of. Cordyceps are a fungus that looks like a mushroom and is known to boost energy, balance blood sugar levels during long bouts of exercise, reduce inflammation, promote kidney function, reduce the risks for type 2 diabetes, and treat erectile dysfunction. Many of these adaptogenic herbs can be taken in pill form or in teas and elixirs. From my experience, I have found them to be effective, beneficial, and are worth trying out for yourself.

100   Choi, B. Y., & Kim, B.-W. (2015) Journal of Cancer Prevention, Withaferin-A Inhibits Colon Cancer Cell Growth by Blocking STAT3 Transcriptional Activity, 20(3), 185–192, http://doi.org/10.15430/JCP.2015.20.3.185

CHAPTER 11
BEAUTY RECIPES

When it comes time to eat, we normally ask ourselves what sounds good or we think about what we are craving. If those foods are fatty, fried, sugary, heavy and starchy, you're not going to feel the love back after you eat them. Perhaps you loathe how you feel after heavy meals and promise to yourself you will start a diet tomorrow. If you battle weight or other issues around food, you may be thinking about what you are going to eat all the time. Perhaps you feel a feeling of anxiety around food which takes the pleasure and joy out of eating. If you are obsessing about food, you may be constantly thinking about how many calories, carbs, and fats you are ingesting, how many cookies you can get away with eating today, or wondering if what you are going to eat will make you break out. Maybe you feel like you don't want to eat anything because you have digestive distress or need to go to the bathroom all the time. This constant mental calculating and guessing around food takes up mental space and can create unnecessary worry. We can't get away from the fact that we need food to survive. I promise, you can do away with dieting forever and eat in abundance, without restriction. It takes a shift in mindset and a few strategy adaptations. Once this occurs, you can enjoy the best foods Earth has and not worry about counting calories, carbs, or fats for the rest of your life. Embrace the phrase: "Eat to live, not live to eat."

Our bodies are designed to run on food as fuel. If you want to look amazing and run at full capacity, you must feed yourself properly. One thing is certain, there is much debate as to which foods are considered "healthy," as dietary theory can be controversial. The foods nobody can argue against are fruits and vegetables. These are beauty foods because they give nutrients like B-complex vitamins, vitamin C, iron, magnesium, phosphorus, potassium, fiber, and flavonoids. Given to us by nature, they combat stress, anxiety, belly bloating, disease, and aging. They promote sleep, stamina, and clear, glowing skin. Purchasing a juicer and a quality blender are great investments to begin with and helps keep juicing affordable. You can purchase one at a time and build up your kitchen tools overtime. Investing in kitchen appliances is investing in your health, and they are your number one health and beauty ally. I use my Vitamix blender and juicer daily. Here are some of the essentials you will want to have in your kitchen: a juicer, blender, food processor, quality knives, spiralizer, cutting board, dehydrator, hand held citrus juicer, and strainer.

Green tea, turmeric, ginger, and lemons are other beauty food powerhouses you want to make a part of your daily routine. Green tea is a great beauty beverage to consume as it is rich in polyphenols, which act like antioxidants, preserving youth. It also has a bit of caffeine in it to give you a little boost. It's not enough caffeine to mess with your cortisol levels, and experts recommend up to three cups of green tea daily. Turmeric also has numerous benefits to sing praises for. It can be used in powder form in recipes, juiced from the root, or taken in pill form. I enjoy juicing it as well as using it in recipes blended with other spices. Studies on turmeric show promising effects on patients with pro-inflammatory diseases like cancers, infections, arthritis, irritable bowel syndrome, psoriasis, cardiovascular disease, diabetes and more.[101]

Ginger and turmeric are in the same family. Ginger is a root that can be juiced or used raw in recipes or salad dressings. Like turmeric, ginger has anti-inflammatory properties and treats ailments like arthritis, indigestion, constipation, ulcers, motion sickness, cardiovascular disorders, vomiting, and diabetes.[102] Ginger is also great for anti-aging because of its antioxidative properties. Stock your kitchen with anti-inflammatory herbs and spices like basil, garlic, pepper, and cinnamon so you will use them in your recipes often. Do not worry if your local grocery store does not carry some of the items you are reading about, like specific supplements, vitamins, sea weeds, hemp seeds, sun dried tomatoes without preservatives, or plant-based protein powders. You can order just about anything for your non-toxic home and personal care items at discounted pricing through Vitacost.com or Amazon. You get free shipping for orders over $50. Thrivemarket.com is also a similar online organic food/home/personal item supplier.

Raw foods feed your inner and outer beauty. Self-image is something people are invested in improving. Plastic surgeons remain in business all to help people improve their outer appearance, and the beauty industry is booming. We seek things that address aging, wrinkles, skin firmness, cellulite, dark circles, puffiness, bloating, strong nails, thick hair, and more. Looking better on the outside does not necessarily change or improve the way we feel on the inside. Feeling good on the inside exudes true beauty and people will be attracted to that. The truth is, we can only do so much on the outside with creams, and makeup is meant to enhance the beauty you already have. The best way to get results is from nourishing yourself from the inside out. Avoid the foods and beverages that will rob you of your beauty and vitality. Yes! This is an inside job.

101   Gupta, S. C., Patchva, S., & Aggarwal, B. B. (2013). Therapeutic Roles of Curcumin: Lessons Learned from Clinical Trials. *The AAPS Journal,* 15(1), 195–218. http://doi.org/10.1208/s12248-012-9432-8

102   Mashhadi, Nafiseh Shokri et al. "Anti-Oxidative and Anti-Inflammatory Effects of Ginger in Health and Physical Activity: Review of Current Evidence." *International Journal of Preventive Medicine* 4.Suppl 1 (2013): S36–S42. Print.

Beauty Nutrients & Food Sources

Nutrients	Food Sources	
Vitamin A: skin firming and smoothing	• Apricots • Cantaloupe • Papaya • Prunes • Asparagus • Broccoli	• Red Pepper • Winter Squashes • Collards Dandelion Greens • Leafy greens • Kale • Spinach
Bioflavonoids	• Apricots • Cherries	• Citrus Fruits Papaya • Buckwheat
Vitamin C: boosts collagen, hydrates skin, skin firming, strengthens immunity	• Tomatoes • Citrus Fruits • Seaweed • Mangoes • Papaya • Alfalfa Sprouts • Pineapple Cantaloupe • Spinach	• Broccoli • Asparagus • Kale • Cauliflower • Kohlrabi • Sauerkraut Cabbage • Leafy Green Vegetables
Biotin: healthy hair, skin, nails, prevents hair loss	• Bananas • Raisins • Almonds • Walnuts	• Legumes • Mushroom • Avocados • Peanuts
Choline B-complex	• Seeds • Nuts • Legumes	• Soy Beans • Green Leafy Vegetables
Folic Acid B-complex	• Cantaloupe • Beets • Cabbage • Asparagus	• Soybeans • Green Leafy Vegetables • Spinach
Inositol B-complex	• Citrus Fruits • Sprouts • Nuts	• Seeds and Spinach • Green Leafy Vegetables
Pantothenic Acid B-complex - great hair	• Cantaloupe • Broccoli • Carrots • Cauliflower • Legumes	• Mushroom • Walnuts • Spinach • Green Leafy Vegetables

Vitamin B1 Thiamine	• Dried Apricots • Avocados • Pineapple • Asparagus • Fresh Peas • Green Leafy Vegetables	• Soybeans • Millet • Sunflower Seeds • Sesame Seeds • Almonds
Vitamin B2 Riboflavin	• Avocados • Broccoli • Asparagus • Okra • Mushroom • Leafy Greens • Spinach	• Kale • Almonds • Soybeans • Lentils • Garbanzos • Buckwheat • Sunflower Seeds
Vitamin B3 Niacin	• Prunes • Dried Figs • Dates • Mushroom • Legumes • Avocados • Asparagus	• Broccoli • Cantaloupe • Millet • Collard Greens • Leafy Greens • Kale • Spinach
Vitamin B6 Pyridoxine	• Raisins • Avocado • Blueberries • Bananas • Cantaloupe	• Cabbage • Mushrooms • Soybeans • Walnuts • Leafy Greens
Vitamin B12, B17	• Sprouts • Sunflower Sprouts	
Vitamin E: Clear skin, anti-inflammatory, powerful antioxidant, fights wrinkles	• Apples • Strawberries • Cherries • Asparagus • Broccoli • Corn • Spinach	• Parsnips • Leeks • Almonds • Green Vegetables • Walnuts • Sunflower Seeds

Protein: builds body cells, good hair health	• Hemp Seeds • Pumpkin Seeds • Chia Seeds • Spinach • Kale • Leafy Greens • Mushrooms • Goji Berries • Maca • Almonds	• Brazil Nuts • Sunflower Seeds • Avocado • Sprouts • Buckwheat • Quinoa • Legumes • Tempeh • Green Peas
Minerals		
Calcium	• Broccoli • Sesame Seeds • Chia Seeds • Almonds • Leafy Green Vegetables • Sunflower Seeds • Kale • Watercress	• Wakame • Hiziki • Collards • Mustard Greens • Dulse • Dandelion Greens • Legumes
Chlorine	• Leafy Greens • Beets • Celery • Carrots	• Onions • Parsnips • Spinach • Dandelion Greens
Chromium	• Leafy Greens • Apples • Raisins • Grapes	• Mushrooms • Legumes • Nuts
Copper	• Cauliflower • Avocado • Almonds • Walnuts • Hazelnuts	• Buckwheat • Millet • Soybeans • Whole Grains
Fluorine	• Brussel Sprouts • Cabbage • Beets • Leafy Greens	• Spinach • Cauliflower • Watercress
Iodine	• Asparagus • Cabbage • Leafy Greens	• Spinach • Cucumbers • Sea Vegetables

Iron	• Dried apricots • Prunes • Spirulina • Raisins • Winter Squashes • Kidney Beans • Brussel Sprouts • Asparagus • Hiziki • Dulse • Leafy Greens	• Kale • Spinach • Millet • Quinoa • Garbanzos • Pumpkin & Sunflower Seeds • Almonds • Cashews • Blackstrap Molasses • Tomato Paste • Sun Dried Tomatoes
Magnesium	• Dried Apricots • Strawberries • Corn • Mushrooms • Swiss Chard • Buckwheat • Millet • Mangoes • Broccoli • Parsnips • Spinach • Soybeans • Wakame	• Avocado • Bananas • Beets • Lentils • Almonds • Dulse • Cantaloupe • Pineapples • Cauliflower • Leafy Greens • Hazelnuts • Pumpkin Seeds
Manganese	• Apples • Apricots • Buckwheat • Celery • Legumes • Almonds	• Pineapples • Bananas • Leafy Greens • Broccoli • Carrots • Hazelnuts
Phosphorus	• Broccoli • Leafy Greens • Dulse • Kale • Garbanzos	• Almonds • Sesame Seeds • Pumpkin Seeds • Collard Greens • Buckwheat
Potassium	• Dates • Bananas • Garlic	• Onion • Cantaloupe • Papaya
Selenium: powerful antioxidants, firms skin, increases elasticity, prevents skin cancer	• Brazil Nuts • Walnuts • Onions	• Whole Grains • Brown Rice

Silicon: strengthens bones, heart, hair, nails, heals skin, benefits digestive system	• Apples • Grapes • Strawberries • Asparagus • Beets	• Celery • Parsnip • Leafy Greens • Spinach • Swiss Chard
Sodium: important electrolyte for cellular activity and the nervous system	• Celery • Leafy Greens • Swiss Chard	• Watercress • Sea Vegetables
Sulphur: firm skin, boosts immunity, healthy joints	• Brussel Sprouts • Cabbage • Celery • Fennel • Bok Choy • Asparagus	• Garlic • Onions • Leafy Greens • Watercress • Swiss Chard
Zinc: shiny healthy hair, clear skin, reduces inflammation, decreases oily skin	• Pumpkin Seeds • Cashews • Mushrooms • Onions • Legumes	• Nuts • Sunflower Seeds • Pumpkin Seeds • Spinach • Green Leafy Vegetables
Essential Fatty Acids: glowing skin, healthy hair, protection from sun damage	• Walnuts • Flax Seeds • Hemp Seeds • Chia Seeds	

Green leafy vegetables cover so many of the essential nutrients our bodies need. They are the foundation for not only a successful plant-based lifestyle, but for your beauty as well. Because green vegetables are so nutrient dense and cleansing, they create an inner glow like no other. To ensure that you get a variety of greens in your diet, be sure to rotate them weekly. Don't just have spinach and romaine lettuce every night in your raw vegetable salad. Mix in some fresh kale, arugula, watercress, sprouts, or other leafy greens as well. Leave off the croutons and top your salad with sprouts or flax crackers instead. You will be happy when you look in the mirror to see how much beauty eating this way gives you. People will want to know what your secret is.

Having the right mindset is important for success because there is no need to let a diet stress you out. Focusing on the positive outcomes of making changes will help you let go of the foods not serving you. Food is a means to fuel and nourish your body, mind, and spirit so you can thrive and express your highest potential. Eating predominantly raw plant foods offers those benefits at the highest level. Eating 100% raw may not be suitable for everybody. Determining that is left up to the individual by experimenting and fine-tuning dietary and energy needs.

Again, there are no hard and fast rules anybody must follow here. It's liberating to know, though, "I can eat whatever I want, but I choose to eat raw foods or vegan foods because they serve me the best." This will keep you out of the restrictive diet trap that people often fall into. If you fall off course and don't like how you feel, just get on course the next time you need to eat, and remember that you are eating to live and not living to eat. Being flexible and allowing yourself to eat cooked foods makes this lifestyle more achievable, especially in social situations. Once you are feeling and looking amazing and up to ten years younger from eating mainly raw foods and juicing, you may find yourself naturally preferring raw. Your quality of life is enhanced the better you eat. Feeding the body poorly, failing to exercise, smoking cigarettes, drinking too much alcohol, and stressing out uncontrollably are taking down lives in large numbers. Many people go to the doctor and end up relying on medications for the rest of their lives. Life threatening diseases are preventable and manageable by following a vegan diet. How much is someone able to enjoy life and help others if they are sick and unwell? We have everything we need to be healed and well already within us. We just need to provide our bodies the proper circumstances for healing to occur. Plug into the miracle and you will feel the difference. Here are some of my favorite recipes I've created and use at home that I'd like to share with you.

Juices

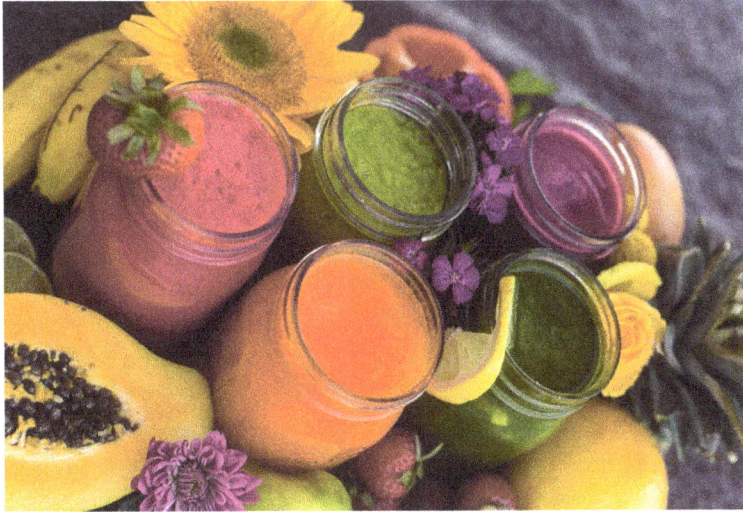

*Note: Adding lemons to your green juice cuts the green taste and makes them taste palatable.

Directions for all Juices:

Wash and cut up the produce if necessary to allow it to fit through your juicer. Run all produce through the juicer and strain off the pulp in a fine mesh strainer. This will make your juice smooth to drink. Enjoy creating beauty juices yourself with some of these recipes as they will feed your health and beauty from the inside out! Aim to get 16-32 oz of fresh juice into your diet often. A 32oz serving is around 1-2 servings.

Green Is the New Pink

Yield: 32 ounces

Ingredients:
1 medium cucumber
1 zucchini
1 lemon (don't have to peel if organic)
6 dinosaur kale leaves
5 celery stalks
2 apples
1-2 inches of ginger

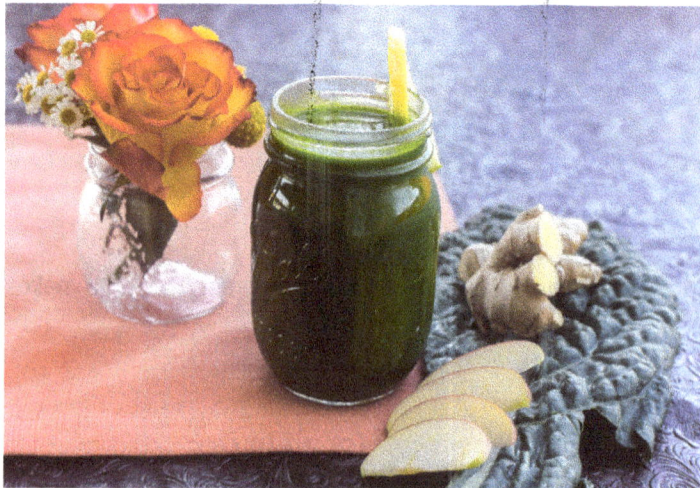

Glowing Beauty Juice 1

Yield: 32 ounces

Ingredients:
6 dinosaur kale leaves
1 lemon
1-2 inches ginger
4 apples (Pink lady apples are my favorite - they are the perfect combo of sweet, crisp, and sour!)
1 medium beet

Glowing Beauty Juice 2

Yield: 32 ounces

Ingredients:
6 dinosaur kale leaves
1 head romaine lettuce
2 apples
1 inch turmeric
2 inches ginger
1 clove garlic
3 celery stalks
1 medium cucumber
1 lemon

Beta C - Mojo Juice

Yield: 1 serving (10oz)

Ingredients:
4 oranges
1 beet

Directions:
Blend the juice with 2 tbsp chia seed, 1 cup of spinach, and 9 ice cubes.
This tastes great ice cold.

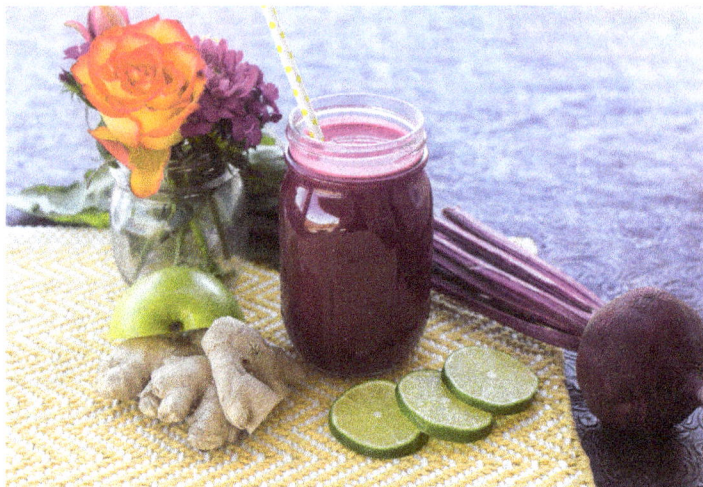

Drop the Beet

Yield: 32 ounces

Ingredients:
¼ small head purple cabbage
1 medium beet
1 lime (trim the peel off before juicing)
3 apples
1-2 inches ginger
1 head romaine lettuce
*Cabbage juice prevents cancer

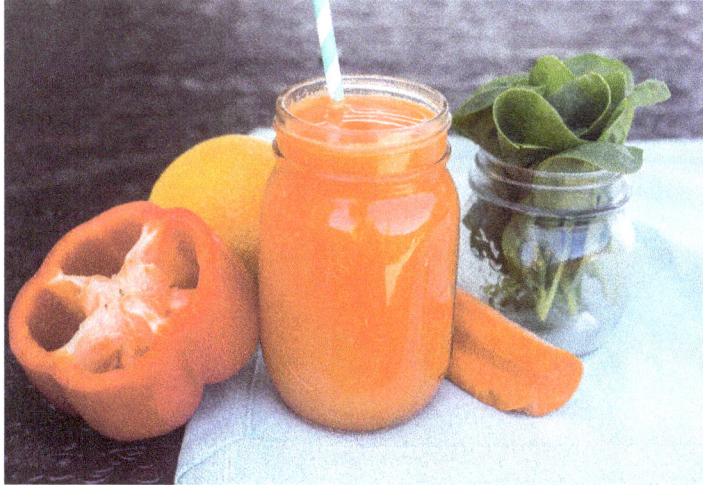

Beta Carotene Blast

Yield: 32 ounces

Ingredients:
4 oranges
4 carrots
1 red pepper
2 inches turmeric

Dance to the Beet

Yield: 32 ounces

Ingredients:
1 beet
2 limes
6 apples
2 inches ginger
2 inches turmeric
½ cup water

Rome If You Want To

Yield: 32 ounces

Ingredients:
1 head romaine lettuce
1-2 inches ginger
 2 inches turmeric
 2 oranges
 2 apples
½ cucumber

The Tom Cat

Yield: 32 ounces

Ingredients:
5 small tomatoes
3 carrots
5 ribs of celery
1 lemon
1 clove garlic
3 cups spinach
1 medium cucumber
Optional: 1 cup parsley

Beautiful Skin Juice

Yield: 32 ounces

Ingredients:
1 sweet potato
1 cucumber
½ pineapple
½ red bell pepper
1 inch of ginger

Shakes and Smoothies

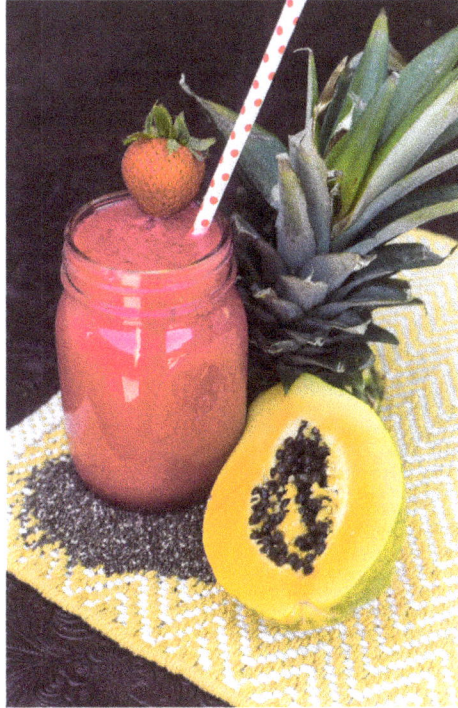

Chocolate Chip Mint Shake

This recipe contains cacao nibs, giving you protein, magnesium, iron, vitamin K, calcium, copper, manganese, potassium, and more. 1 tbsp boosts 12mg of natural caffeine, and these are a great alternative to chocolate chips because they don't contain any sugar!

Yield: 1 serving

Ingredients:
2 tbsp cacao nibs
¼ tsp peppermint extract
¼ tsp vanilla extract
1 scoop of chocolate plant-based protein powder
1 cup frozen banana
 5-6 ice cubes
1.5 cups filtered water or unsweetened hemp milk or almond milk

*Option 1: add 1 cup raw spinach or kale for added nutrition and fiber.

*Option 2: add 2 tbsp Irish sea moss gel for a hair, skin, and nail booster!

*Option 3: add 1 tsp of maca powder for a turbocharged boost.
You can add all the above.

Directions:
Blend the ingredients in a high-speed blender (except the cacao nibs) until large chunks are smooth. Then add the nibs and blend again for a few more seconds. This tastes just like an ice cream shake and will make you feel great!

Cashew Cinnamon Dream Nut Milk

Yield: 1 serving

Ingredients:
¼ cup soaked cashews
½ tsp cinnamon
2-3 pitted dates
1 tsp vanilla
6 ice cubes
2 cups water
*Creamy mineral rich option: add 1 tbsp of Irish sea moss.

Directions:
Add all ingredients into the blender and blend until creamy and smooth. Enjoy!

Vanilla Cashew Nut Milk

Yield: 3 cups

Ingredients:
1 cup soaked cashews
¼ cup coconut palm sugar
½ tbsp vanilla
4 cups cold water

Directions:
Blend all the ingredients in the blender for up to 60 seconds and strain through a nut milk bag. Store in the refrigerator for up to one week.

Almond Date Nut Milk

Yield: 28 ounces

Ingredients:
1 cup soaked almonds
4 pitted dates
Pinch of sea salt
1 tsp vanilla extract (optional)
4 cups water

Directions:
Blend almonds, salt, and dates in the blender until smooth. Then strain the mixture through a nut milk bag. This is a delicious sweet milk and is perfect to add to matcha or English Breakfast tea for added flavor and creaminess. You can also bake with this and it tastes delicious because it is homemade! To give the milk a holiday flair, add 1 tsp pumpkin spice to the mixture.

Seize the Day Smoothie

Yield: 1 serving (12 oz)

Ingredients:
1 frozen banana (approximately 1 cup)
5-6 frozen strawberries
1 cup cold vanilla cashew milk (see my recipe)
½ cup coconut water
½ cup raw spinach
Optional: 1 tsp spirulina

Directions:
Place all ingredients in a high-speed blender and blend for 30-60 seconds until smooth.

Orange Spinach Basil Smoothie

Yield: 1-2 servings

Ingredients:
32 ounces fresh orange juice (6-8 oranges)
2 cups of spinach
½ cup fresh basil
1.5 cups ice

Directions:
First, juice the oranges and pour the juice into a blender. Next, add in the spinach and ice cubes. Blend for 30-60 seconds, then add the basil. Blend for a few more seconds. The bright flavors of this smoothie are sure to brighten your day and make you feel amazing!

Double Chocolate Mint Mocha Smoothie

Yield: 1 serving (16 oz)

Ingredients:
1 frozen banana
1 scoop chocolate plant-based protein powder
1 cup raw spinach
½ tsp vanilla
¼ teaspoon mint extract
2 tbsp Dandy Blend
1 tbsp cacao powder
1 cup water or coconut water
6 ice cubes

Directions:
Add ingredients into your blender and blend until smooth. This is by far my favorite smoothie. Dandy Blend adds a coffee-like flavor but doesn't contain any caffeine. It is a great coffee alternative and is made with dandelion, which is detoxifying for your liver.

Chocolate Cherry Smoothie

Yield: 1 serving

Ingredients:
1 cup frozen banana
½ cup frozen pitted cherries
1 scoop chocolate plant-based protein powder
1 cup water or (your favorite plant-based milk)
1 tsp almond butter
1 cup ice

Directions:
Fill your blender with ice and the smoothie ingredients. Blend it all well until smooth and frosty. This is a great smoothie to have if you are having a sweet craving because it is sweet, chocolatey, filling, and satisfying.

Orange Banana Smoothie

Yield: 1 serving

Ingredients:
2 whole oranges, peeled
1 frozen banana
1 cup water or cashew milk
1 tsp vanilla
1 tsp spirulina powder
4-5 ice cubes

Directions:
Blend her up and drink her down!

Love Life Smoothie

Yield: 1 serving

Ingredients:
2 frozen bananas
½ cup frozen blueberries
4 frozen strawberries
1 cup raw spinach
1 date
1 tsp almond butter
1 cup water
4 ice cubes
1 tsp vanilla extract

Directions:
Blend the ingredients together for 30-60 seconds until smooth and top with 1 tsp of chia seeds.

Glowing Smoothie

Yield: 32 ounces

Ingredients:
Juice ½ pineapple
½ large cucumber
1 orange
5 celery ribs
1 lemon
1 lime
1.5 cups ice

Directions:
First, juice the produce and strain. Then blend the juice with 1 cup of spinach and 1 tbsp of chia seeds with for added protein and omega-3 fatty acids. Blend in the ice for a cold, frosty finish.

Strawberry Cream Dream Smoothie

Yield: 1 serving

Ingredients:
1 cup vanilla plant-based milk
5 ice cubes
2 pitted dates
1 banana
6 frozen strawberries
Optional beauty boost: 1 tbsp Irish sea moss gel
1 tsp chia seeds

Directions:
Place all ingredients in a high-speed blender and mix it up until smooth. This smoothie is so satisfying and delicious. It's perfect for breakfast, a snack, or even dessert! Yum!

Morning Sunshine Smoothie

Yield: 1 serving

Ingredients:
1 frozen banana
½ cup frozen mango
4 frozen strawberries
1 cup coconut water
4 ice cubes

Directions:
Blend until smooth and light up the day! You are beautiful!

Acai Bowl

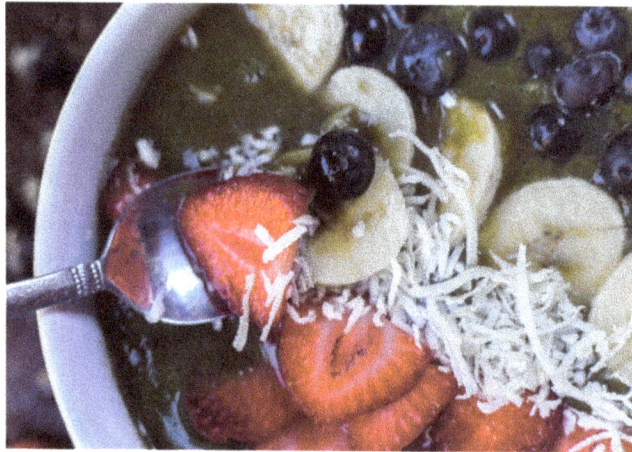

Yield: 1 serving

Let me tell you why you will love this recipe: It makes you feel great, and acai berries have the highest levels of antioxidants out of all berries! This anti-aging concoction is energizing and can help you fight off a cold. There have been times I have come home after a long day of work, feeling tired and drained. Instead of slamming down an energy drink or cup of coffee to power through an evening workout, I ate a homemade acai bowl and felt instantly energized and rejuvenated. These are great as pre or post workout meals. Any time of the day is a good time for an acai bowl. The health and beauty benefits are long-term. The acai looks green in this photo because the packets of acai used had greens in them. Usually, acai is a deep berry purple color.

Ingredients:
2 packets of frozen unsweetened acai
½ cup or more of apple juice (to get the consistency you desire)
1 frozen banana
¼ cup sliced strawberries
¼ cup blueberries
2 tbsp shredded coconut
*Sprinkle chia seeds on top for a healthy dose of protein and omega fatty acids.

Directions:
Blend frozen acai, apple juice, and banana together to make the frozen base. You can use your choice of plant-based milk instead of apple juice if you want. Alternatively, you can blend in your choice of favorite frozen fruits with banana to the acai base to change it up. Fruits that work well mixed into the base include bananas, strawberries, blueberries, pineapple, and mango. Get creative and experiment with the acai blend fruit combos for fun. Next, pour the frozen base into a bowl and top with fresh fruit, like strawberries, avocado, blueberries, sliced banana, figs, shredded coconut, chia seeds, chopped nuts, grain-free granola, nut butter, or whatever kinds of toppings you want.

I highly recommend adding some superfood goodness to your bowl to kick up the health and beauty benefits into high gear! Some options are:

- Pomegranate powder

- Goji berries, maca powder, spirulina, chia seeds, or cacao nibs

- Hemp seeds, which contain protein and omega fatty acids for hormonal and brain health (Remember: your body needs fat to flourish.)

Entrees

Broccoli Sun-Dried Tomato Pâté

Yield: 3 cups

Ingredients:
1 cup broccoli florets
1 cup cauliflower florets
1 clove garlic
6 soaked sun-dried tomatoes (about ¼ cup)
½ cup ground flax seeds
½ cup chopped green onion
3 tbsp coconut aminos
3 tbsp tahini
Juice of 1 lemon
*Fresh herbs, like rosemary, oregano, thyme and/or parsley, to taste

Directions:
Pulse the broccoli and cauliflower in a food processor to "rice" it. You may need to scrape down the sides and pulse again and again to get it finely chopped. Add the rest of the ingredients and continue to process until well combined. You can use this pâté to fill collard wraps and lettuce leaves or to form patties and dehydrate to make burgers. Delish!

Carrot Pumpkin Seed Pâté

Yield: 2-3 cups

Ingredients:
6 sundried tomatoes, soaked
½ cup pumpkin seeds, soaked
1 tsp sesame oil
1 garlic clove
1 date
6 carrots, peeled and sliced into small pieces
1 tsp raw ginger chopped
1 tsp rice wine vinegar or apple cider vinegar

Directions:
Add all ingredients in the food processor and blend it until a chunky yet sticky consistency is accomplished. Use this pâté in sushi rolls, collard wraps, or inside lettuce leaves.

Bowl Chili

Yield: approximately 5 cups

Ingredients:
5 cups diced tomatoes
½ cup red pepper, chopped
½ cup green onions, sliced
¾ cup fresh cilantro, chopped
1 avocado, diced
1 jalapeno pepper, seeded
2 cups mushrooms
½ cup sundried tomatoes
2 tsp fresh lemon juice
3 tsp chili powder
1 tsp cumin
1 clove garlic
½ cup soaked walnuts or pumpkin seeds
½ cup water

Directions:
Clean and prep the vegetables. First, create the chili base. In a blender, add the sundried tomatoes, garlic, lemon juice, fresh tomatoes, chili powder, cumin, and jalapeno. Blend for up to a minute, then add the walnuts, mushrooms, and water. Blend a bit more until a smooth but chunky texture is achieved. Pour the mixture into a bowl and mix in the rest of the ingredients. Serve with sliced radishes, raw crackers, organic corn chips, a side salad, brown rice, or quinoa.

Collard Green Vegetable Beauty Wraps

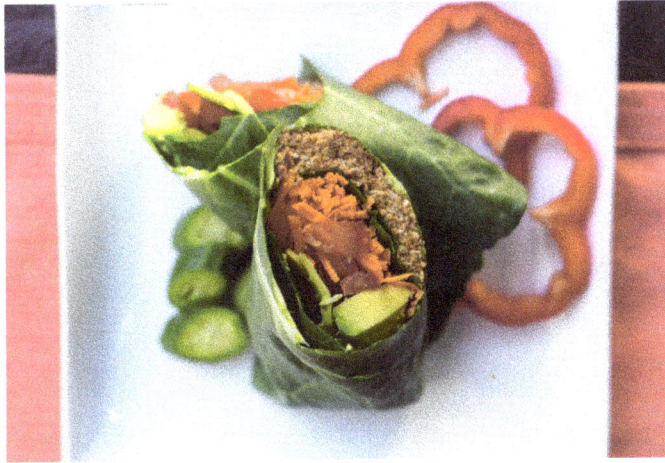

Yield: 1 bunch of collard greens serves 2-3

Collard leaves are 20% protein, contain B-vitamins, thiamin, riboflavin, and niacin!

*Use them in place of bread and fill them up with your choice of filling, whether it be a pâté or "burger." Soak the leaves in hot water for a few minutes to wash and soften up before drying them off and rolling them up. Choose your other favorite fillings, like sprouts, romaine lettuce, sliced bell peppers, red onion, Kalamata olives, avocado, cucumber, mango, shredded carrots, or sliced tomato.

Directions:
Run a knife over the thick stem of the collard leaf to thin it down and make it more pliable. Place your favorite fillings near one end, fold in the sides of the leaf and roll it up. Eat it like that or cut it in half for smaller pieces. These store well in the fridge and are easy to make ahead of time for grabbing and eating on the go.

Collard wraps contain Vitamin K. This vitamin not only protects your heart, builds bones, and helps control blood sugar levels, it also prevents some cancers and Alzheimer's disease. Most people are deficient in this vitamin. These are great reasons to eat collard wraps!

Zucchini Noodles

Yield: 2 servings

Ingredients:
4 zucchinis
4 tomatoes
½ cup sundried tomatoes
1 date
1 clove garlic
Crushed red pepper flakes, to taste
6 fresh basil leaves

Directions:
Spiralize the zucchini into noodles or shred them with a food processor and set aside in a bowl. Next, blend the rest of the ingredients, except the basil, in a blender until well combined. Add the basil in last and pulse a few times to chop it into the sauce. Finally, pour the sauce onto the noodles and enjoy!

Shredded Yam Salad

Yield: 1 serving
1 raw yam, shredded or spiralized
1 zucchini, shredded or spiralized
2 carrots, shredded
2-3, tbsp pumpkin seeds
2 tbsp minced red onions
¼ cup papaya, diced
1-2 tbsp hemp seeds
Sesame ginger dressing

Directions:
Wash and peel the yam and either shred it with a food processor or noodle it with a spiralizer. Do the same with the zucchini. You do not have to peel it as a lot of nutrition is in the green skin. Shred the carrots as well. In your bowl, add the yams, zucchini, carrots, and papaya. Top this salad with the rest of the ingredients, including the dressing, and enjoy. You will feel energized and light after eating this!

Kelp Noodle Pad Thai

Yield: 1-2 servings

Ingredients:
1 package raw kelp noodles
1 red bell pepper
½ cup carrots, chopped or shredded
¾ cup green sprouts (sunflower, broccoli)
3 green onion sprigs
1 tsp mint, chopped
1 tbsp fresh basil, chopped
1 tbsp fresh cilantro
1 cup cucumber, diced
Sesame ginger dressing

Directions:
Rinse and soak the kelp noodles in hot water with the juice of a lemon for 30 minutes (this will soften the noodles) while you prep the vegetables and sauce. In the meantime, chop up the bell pepper, cucumber, mint, basil, and cilantro. Slice up the green onion and shred the carrots. Prepare the sauce in a blender, and when done, drain the noodles and dry them off with a towel. Next, put them in a large bowl and top with the other fresh vegetables. Pour the dressing on top and toss all together to cover the noodles. If you want the noodles even softer, let them sit for up to 15 minutes. Garnish with sprouts and avocado and enjoy! This is so good!

The All-American Beet Burger

Yield: 2 servings

Ingredients:
3 cups raw beets, shredded
2 cloves garlic
½ cup soaked raw pumpkin seeds
½ cup soaked sundried tomatoes
Juice of 1 lemon
½ cup nutritional yeast
3 tsp fennel seeds
2 tsp mustard powder
1 tsp sea salt
1 cup flax meal
2 tbsp tahini

Directions:
Process ingredients in a food processor until smooth. Scoop out the batter and form patties 4 inches in diameter on dehydrator sheets. Dehydrate for 6-8 hours at 115-118°F, flipping them over half way through the full length of time. Finally, wrap these up in collard leaves with red onion, avocado and sprouts, or sandwich them between romaine lettuce leaves. These burgers are so good, you won't be able to eat just one at a time. At least, I can't!

Sunshine Patty

Yield: 2 servings

I am amazed at how much this recipe has the taste and texture of Thanksgiving stuffing! It's DELICIOUS, and can be eaten as-is or formed into patties and dehydrated to make burgers. You are going to love this!

Ingredients:
2 cups zucchini, shredded
½ cup soaked sunflower seeds
3 tbsp tahini
½ cup sundried tomatoes
2 garlic cloves
½ cup green onions
3 tbsp fresh dill, chopped
Juice of ½ lemon
½ cup carrot, shredded
1 tsp mustard powder
½ cup psyllium husk
3 tbsp fresh parsley
½ cup celery
Salt and pepper, to taste

Directions:
First shred the carrots and zucchini. Then add the rest of the ingredients in a food processor. Process for a few seconds. Then, scrape down the sides and add the psyllium husk. Process again to combine well and scoop out to form patties around 3 inches in diameter. Dehydrate for 4-6 hours at 115°F.

Sauces and Dressings

Sweet Avocado Curry

Yield: 2.5 cups

Ingredients:
2 cups fresh mango
5 sun dried tomatoes (¼ cup)
½ tsp chili flakes
½ cup avocado
½ cup carrot, peeled and chopped
1 tsp sesame oil
1 tsp curry powder
¼ cup fresh lemon juice
¼ cup water or more for desired consistency

Directions:
Blend up the ingredients in a high-speed blender until smooth. This dressing rocks over kelp noodles with spinach, sliced carrots, red cabbage, and sprouts. You will love this!

Tangy Island Dressing

Yield: 2 cups

Ingredients:
1 cup fresh mango
¼ cup fresh lemon juice
1.5 cups fresh tomatoes, diced
½ tsp Ume plum vinegar
2 tbsp jalapeno, seeded and chopped
⅓ cup green onion, chopped

Directions:
Place all ingredients in a high-speed blender and blend for 30 seconds until smooth.

Creamy Garlic Sauce

Yield: 1 cup

Ingredients:
1 cup raw cashews (soaked, if possible)
¼ cup lemon
1 clove garlic
1 cup or more of water to reach desired consistency
¼ tsp sea salt
3 tbsp nutritional yeast
For a yummy variation, add 2 tbsp sundried tomatoes

Directions:
Add ingredients into the blender and blend well until smooth and creamy.

Original Vegan Ranch

Yield: 10 ounces

Ingredients:
1 cup soaked cashews
¼ cup fresh lemon juice
2 tbsp fresh dill
2 tbsp fresh parsley
1 tbsp chives
1 clove garlic
¼ tsp sea salt
3/4 cup water
Optional: ½ tsp black pepper

Directions:
Add ingredients in the blender and blend until creamy.

Creamy Cilantro Dressing

Yield: 1 cup

Ingredients:
1 cup cashews (soaked, if possible)
1 clove garlic
Juice of 1 lemon (about ¼ cup)
3/4 cup water
½ cup fresh cilantro
Salt, to taste

Directions:
Add all ingredients in your blender, except the cilantro, and blend until creamy and smooth. Finally, add the cilantro and blend for 10 more seconds.

Vegan Caesar Dressing

Yield: 1 cup

Ingredients:
½ cup soaked cashews
¼ cup olive oil
¾ cup celery
Juice of 1 lemon (around ¼ cup)
2 tbsp nutritional yeast
1 tsp mustard powder
4 tsp capers
2 cloves of garlic
½ tsp sea salt
½ tsp black pepper
⅓ cup filtered water or more to reach your desired consistency

Directions:
Add all ingredients in the blender and blend well.

Sesame Ginger Sauce

Yield: 14 ounces

Ingredients:
1 whole orange, peeled
1 date
Juice of 1 lemon (¼ cup)
1 clove garlic
1 tbsp almond butter
1 tbsp raw tahini
2 tbsp coconut aminos or ¼ tsp sea salt
1 tsp sesame oil
2 tsp fresh ginger, peeled and chopped
½ tbsp raw apple cider vinegar
½ cup water
Optional: 1 tbsp chopped jalapeno pepper or 1 tsp crushed red pepper flakes

Directions:
Blend these ingredients up until smooth. This sauce is amazing, and can be used for noodles, salad dressing, or as a dipping sauce.

Succulent Salads

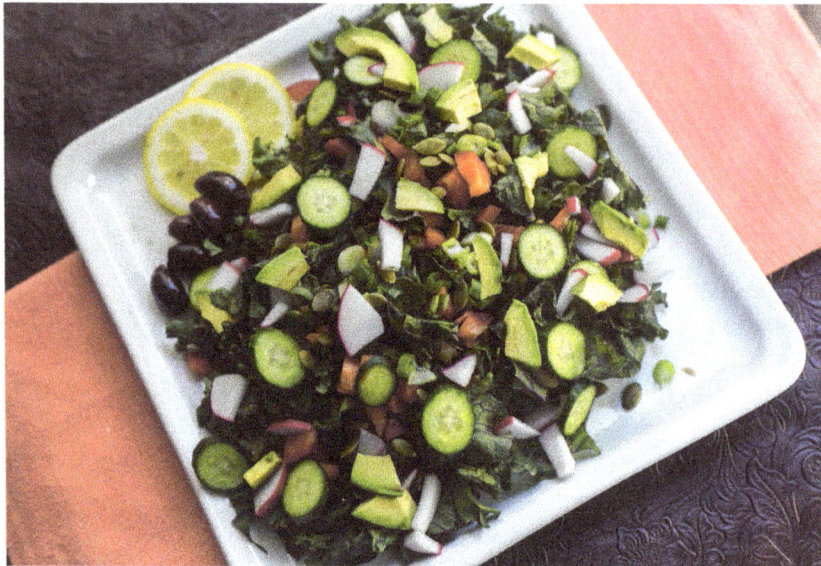

You Are Strong

Yield: 2-4 servings

Ingredients:
1 head kale (approximately 6-7 cups), massaged
Wash, dry, and massage the kale for around 3 minutes, until soft and tender. This tenderizes the kale. Then, add the spinach and the rest of the ingredients.
2 packed cups raw spinach
1.5 cups radishes, chopped
1 cup cucumber, chopped
1 cup kalamata olives
½ cup dried currants
Black pepper, to taste
1 avocado (1 cup chopped)
¼ cup lemon zest

Lemon Vinaigrette Dressing

Yield: 1 cup

Ingredients:
½ cup olive oil
⅓ cup fresh lemon juice
2 tbsp coconut sugar
3 tbsp apple cider vinegar.
Top with fresh herbs, like organic dill, parsley or cilantro.

I could eat a kale salad for dinner literally every night, and sometimes I do. It never gets old because I change it up with different dressings and veggie combinations. Kale contains zinc, B vitamins, vitamin E, lutein, and zeaxanthin, which keeps your vision healthy. Kale also contains compounds called glucosinolates, and once those compounds are chewed, they prevent growth of cancer cells.

Killin' It Kale Salad

Yield: 7 cups

Ingredients:
1 head of massaged curly kale
*You can add other greens, like spinach, romaine, or arugula.
1 avocado
4 tbsp olive oil
Juice of 1 lemon
½ cup Kalamata olives
2 tbsp hemp seeds
1 cup radishes, washed and sliced
½ cup diced tomato
3 tbsp pumpkin seeds
¼ cup parsley

Directions:
Add ingredients to your bowl and use the lemon and olive oil as a dressing!

Poppin' Chili Dill Salad

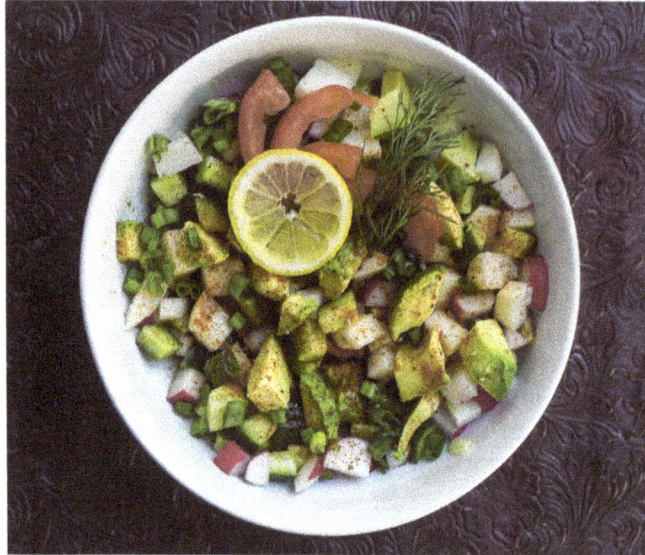

Yield: 1 serving

Ingredients:
1 cucumber
4 radishes
1 cup jicama
1 avocado
½ cup green onions
½ cup fresh dill
juice of ½ - 1 lemon, to taste
1 tsp chili powder
Sea salt, to taste

Directions:
Peel the jicama and cucumber. Leave some of the skin on the cucumber since it contains vitamins and minerals, like calcium, phosphorus, potassium, sodium, vitamin C, magnesium, and B-complex. Cucumbers are hydrating and rejuvenating. Chop and dice the vegetables and place them in a bowl. Squeeze the lemon juice on top of the medley and add the chili and salt. Toss the salad together and coat all the pieces.

The Peacemaker

Yield: 1-2 servings

Ingredients:
½ cup sundried tomatoes
1.5 cups cauliflower rice
1 tablespoon hemp seeds
2 cups kale, chopped
¼ cup Kalamata olives
Juice ½ lemon
½ avocado
2 tbsp currants
Salt and pepper, to taste
Pine nut pesto*

Directions:
In a food processor, rice a head of cauliflower by placing chopped pieces in the container with the S-blade. You may have to stop processing a few times to scrape down the sides, and then reprocess to get it all into little pieces. Scoop out half of the contents and add the sundried tomatoes. Continue to process until well combined. Mix the sundried tomato mixture with enough rice to make around 2 cups. Next, chop up some green curly kale and measure up 2 cups. Put that in a large bowl and place 2 cups of the cauliflower mixture on top. Sprinkle on the currants, olives, avocado, and hemp seeds as well. Squeeze some fresh lemon juice on top and mix it all together. The pine nut pesto tastes great on top of this salad. Mix it all up and dive in!

Pine Nut Pesto*

Yield: 1 cup

Ingredients:
½ cup pine nuts
½ cup parsley
½ cup basil
2 cloves garlic
2 tbsp lemon juice
1 cup zucchini, sliced
¼ tsp sea salt

Directions:
Place your ingredients in a food processor and pulse with the S-blade until well combined. You can also use your blender if you desire. Use this to flavor salads and dishes such as pastas, zucchini noodles, or as a sandwich spread. Yum!

Vegan Sushi

Now swim with me as we dive into raw vegan sushi recipes. Let's take a moment to discuss why seaweed is important to incorporate into your diet. Seaweed is an incredible beauty food. These ocean plants are fantastic health foods, and you may need to acquire a taste for them. Seaweed has both high protein and mineral contents. They also contain iodine, calcium, magnesium, and more vitamin C than oranges. Natural iodine helps thyroid function and has other benefits. Seaweeds help stabilize blood sugar, improve liver function, have antibacterial, antiviral and anti-inflammatory properties. They are also great for the skin, hair, and nails. Varieties include kelp, hijiki, wakame, dulse, and Irish sea moss.

Irish sea moss is rich in collagen, which boosts skin firmness and elasticity. I highly recommend using Irish sea moss for many reasons. Nutritionally, it contains fiber, protein, Vitamin A, potassium, and iron. Other benefits of Irish sea moss include antimicrobial and antiviral properties, mild laxative effects, digestive soothing, and mucous dissolution. Once the moss is rinsed, soaked, and blended with water, it has a firm, gel-like consistency, and is tasteless. It takes on the flavors of whatever it's being combined with. You can make desserts with it, thicken soups, make cheeses, or add it to smoothies. I personally love using it! Other seaweeds can be sprinkled in salads, mixed in soups, or used to make sushi. I used to love eating sushi with raw fish, but once I learned about parasites and the multitudes of microscopic eggs nestled inside the raw fish, I was DONE. No worms for me, thank you. Without further ado, let's make some vegan sushi.

Raw Vegan Sushi Rolls

Yield: 2 servings

Ingredients:
2-3 sheets nori
Fresh mango slices
Cucumber, sliced into thin strips
Avocado slices
Carrot sesame ginger pâté
Sunflower sprouts
Romaine lettuce

Directions:
On a bamboo sushi mat, lay out a nori sheet and evenly spread the carrot sesame ginger pâté on it. About 2 inches in from the edge of the nori sheet, arrange the romaine lettuce, avocado, mango, cucumber, and sunflower sprouts across the width of the nori. Then, fold it over and roll it up tightly. Once the nori soaks up some of the moisture and seals up, take it out, and slice it into bite-sized chunks with a sharp knife. Dip it in coconut aminos mixed with wasabi and top with pickled ginger if you want an authentic sushi flavor. These rolls are so delicious!

Mushroom Sushi Rolls

Yield: 3 rolls

Ingredients:
1 cup "riced" cauliflower
1 cucumber, sliced into strips
1 avocado, sliced
1 cup marinated chopped mushrooms
1 carrot, thinly sliced
3 nori sheets
Sprouts
Sesame ginger dipping sauce

Directions:
In a bowl, marinate the mushrooms in 1 tsp sesame oil, 1 tsp coconut aminos, and 1 tsp lemon juice. Set aside for 20 minutes. Take a nori sheet and lay it over the bamboo mat shiny side down. Spread 1/3 cup riced cauliflower over the nori to cover it well. On the edge nearest you, lay out the cucumber, avocado, mushrooms, carrots, and sprouts horizontally from side to side. Then, take the top of the nori mat and roll it over tightly and keep rolling as you tuck the ingredients in. Press it all together firmly until the moisture seals the nori. Take your roll out and slice it into bite-sized sushi chunks (4-6 pieces).

Desserts

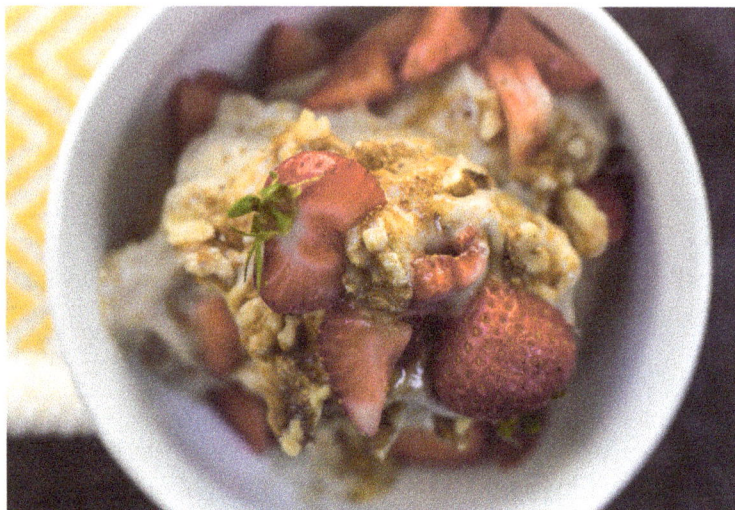

Did you remember to save room? For what, you ask? Dessert! After all, this is what we are saving room for, right? All too often, dieting can make people feel as if dessert is a guilty pleasure. Making delicious desserts with whole, fresh ingredients is the key to having your cake and eating it too. These recipes contain no processed sugars and the sweeteners I recommend using are dates, coconut nectar, palm coconut sugar, and stevia.

Maple syrup and agave nectar are good to use in moderation. Grade B maple syrup is higher in nutrition than Grade A. Discovering your glucose tolerance and experimenting with different natural vegan sweeteners is helpful to see which ones work best for you. Note: When using dates in your recipes, they should be soft. If they are not, soak them in warm water for 20 minutes until they moisten up for better blending.

Dark chocolate is a health and beauty friendly treat, high in antioxidants and mood boosting elements. Aim for the 70-80% chocolate varieties, as they are low in sugar, and you can even find them sweetened with stevia. This type of dark chocolate gives you a healthy dose of antioxidants. Of course, with dessert, fat and calories still add up whether they are healthy or not, so remember to consume in moderation. The great thing about raw vegan desserts is they are the most guilt-free of all desserts and you still feel great after eating them!

Banana Nice Cream Sundae

Yield: 1 serving

Ingredients:
4-6 frozen bananas
1 tsp vanilla extract

Directions:
Blend the bananas and vanilla in a high-speed blender until a frozen yogurt-like consistency is reached. You can add a little water to facilitate blending if necessary. Scoop out the nice cream into a bowl and top with some of your favorite sundae toppers. Prepare to fall in love!

Topping recommendations: sliced strawberries, chopped nuts, dates, almond butter, cacao nibs, goji berries.

Strawberry Banana "Fro-Yo"

Yield: 1 serving

Ingredients:
4-6 frozen bananas
1 cup frozen strawberries
¼ cup coconut water or plain water to facilitate blending

Directions:
Chop the bananas in large chunks and blend up in a high-speed blender until the mixture has a fro-yo-like consistency and scoop it out into a bowl. Top with your favorite toppings, if you please, and dig in.

Apple Banana Bowl

Yield: 1 serving

Ingredients:
1 apple, chopped
1 banana, sliced
3 dates, diced
Cinnamon, to taste

Directions:
Place the chopped apple, banana, and dates in a bowl. Then sprinkle with cinnamon to taste. Top with 1 tsp almond butter or 3 tbsp chopped pecans, cacao nibs, and coconut flakes. Pour your favorite plant-based milk over the top and eat like a breakfast cereal.

Chocolate Orange Cake

Yield: One 9-inch pie

For the crust:
1 cup almonds
1 cup pecans
½ cup dates, pitted
½ cup mulberries, dried
½ cup cacao powder
2 tbsp coconut nectar
¼ tsp sea salt

For the top layer:
½ cup soaked cashews
¾ cup avocado
4 dates
½ cup Irish sea moss
8 oz cup freshly squeezed orange juice

Directions:
Place the crust ingredients in a food processor with the S blade. If the dough is too crumbly, add 1 tbsp of water until it comes together. Press the dough down in a pie dish and set aside. Next, blend the top layer ingredients in a high-speed blender and pour on top of the chocolate crust. Set the cake in the refrigerator to set up. Have a slice and be sure to share with your loved ones!

Spice Up Your Life Truffles

Yield: 16 truffles

Ingredients:
1.5 cups soft dates
½ cup cacao powder
½ cup pecans or almonds
3 tbsp coconut butter
¼ cup goji berries or dried apricots (unsulphured)
¼ tsp cayenne powder
1 tbsp maca powder
¼ teaspoon sea salt

Directions:
Place all the ingredients into a high-speed blender and blend until the contents are chopped down. Next, scoop down the sides and repeat to get everything processed and combined to make the batter stick together. Then, scoop out a tbsp of dough and press in your hands, rolling into a truffle ball. Once you have gone through all the batter, place the truffles on a pan and into the freezer to set. You can dip them in Magic Chocolate Sauce* and roll in hemp seeds with a dash of sea salt and cacao nibs. The chocolate will get hard with the hemp/cacao bits mixed in, providing a bit of a crunch. You can also just roll them in hemp seeds without the chocolate sauce or leave them as-is! Place the finished truffles in an airtight container and store either in the fridge or the freezer. These are so good! They are rich, decadent, and satisfying!

Chocolate Covered Banana Bites

Yield: 2-3 bananas

Ingredients:
Frozen banana chunks, sliced ½-inch thick
2 tbsp hemp seeds
2 tbsp cacao nibs
⅛ tsp sea salt

Directions:
Take some ripe, spotted bananas and peel them. Slice them up into bite-sized chunks. Next, place them in a Ziploc bag and pop them into the freezer to harden up. Have some Magic Chocolate Sauce handy in a bowl (see my recipe*) and mix in 2 tbsp each of hemp seeds and cacao nibs. These ingredients give the bites a crunchy texture within the chocolate that is reminiscent of a Nestlé crunch bar. Once frozen, dip each banana bite in the chocolate sauce mixture until covered. The chocolate sauce should harden right away over the frozen banana. Eat them immediately or pop them in a container and store in the freezer. You are going to love these!

Magic Chocolate Sauce*

Yield: approximately ½ cup

Ingredients:
½ cup coconut oil
1 tsp vanilla extract
2 tbsp coconut nectar
2 tbsp cacao powder

Directions:
You will want your coconut oil to be in a liquid state. If it's not, place the jar in a pot of hot water to warm it up and liquify the oil. Then, mix all the ingredients together in a bowl and enjoy this as a chocolate fondue type of sauce. Dip strawberries, bananas, berries, or pick your favorite fruit to cover in chocolate sauce and devour! If the fruit is frozen, the sauce will harden and become a chocolatey frozen treat.

Raspberry Cheesecake

Yield: One 9-inch pie pan

For the filling:
½ cup soaked pine nuts
½ cup Irish sea moss gel
¾ cup avocado
½ cup lemon juice
2 tbsp coconut oil
½ cup coconut nectar

For the glaze:
1 cup raspberries
6 soaked dates
2 tbsp Irish sea moss gel
1 tbsp coconut nectar

For the crust:
8 soft dates, pitted
1 cup pecans
1 cup almonds
½ cup dried mulberries
2 tbsp coconut nectar
1 tsp vanilla
¼ tsp salt

Directions:
Soak the pine nuts in water for 2 hours or overnight, which is optional. Start by making the crust. Combine the crust ingredients in a food processor and combine them until the mixture comes together well. Spread the dough in a springboard pie pan. Put that in the refrigerator. Next, combine the filling ingredients in a blender and process until smooth. Pour this mixture on top of the crust and set back into the refrigerator. Make a raspberry glaze by blending the raspberries, dates, and other ingredients together until smooth. Pour this on top of the filling and spread evenly for the top layer. Place the pie back in the freezer for a few hours to set. Before serving, allow it to thaw out a little bit. This is a perfect dessert to share at a BBQ or holiday gathering. Your friends and family will love this! Knowing it does the body good makes it even better!

Who doesn't LOVE chocolate? Raw organic cacao powder is full of antioxidants and is a good source of magnesium, protein, and iron. It also contains calcium and potassium. Take your smoothies to the next level and add 2 tbsp of cacao powder to the mix and boost your health and beauty! This next recipe is chock-full of raw cacao powder and is made from fresh, whole foods.

Fudgy Brownies

Yield: One 8 or 9-inch pan

Ingredients:
2 cups dates, pitted
⅓ cup cacao powder
1 cup almonds or pecans
1 tsp vanilla
¼ tsp sea salt
3 tbsp water
Optional: add 1 tsp maca powder and 1-2 tsp cayenne powder to kick these brownies up a notch!

Directions:
First, process the nuts in a food processor to grind them into a flour and then combine with chopped dates, cacao, vanilla, and sea salt. Add the water to the mixture to moisten it up. The batter should form together to make a dough and not be too crumbly. Line an 8x8 baking pan with plastic wrap or parchment paper. Place the dough into the pan and press it down evenly. Let it set in the fridge while you make the frosting.

Chocolate Avocado Frosting

Yield: 2 cups

Ingredients:
2 large avocados (about 2 cups)
6 pitted dates (about ½ cup - it's best to soak the dates for 30 minutes in hot water to soften them up for easy blending)
2 tbsp maple syrup or coconut nectar
½ tsp vanilla extract
⅔ cup cacao powder

Directions:
For the frosting, put all the ingredients in a blender and blend it until smooth and creamy. You will need to pause blending and scrape down the sides a few times to get everything combined. Spread the frosting over the brownie batter, cover with plastic wrap and put it back in the fridge to set up. Then take them out and slice them up. These are rich and fudgy, and they pair great with fresh berries and mint.

CHAPTER 12

MOVEMENT FOR PHYSICAL AND MENTAL WELLNESS

All the recipes in this book are life-giving and promote a clean body and mind. The food we eat and our movement, or lack thereof, affects the way we think and feel. Therefore, exercise is a key component to a healthy lifestyle.

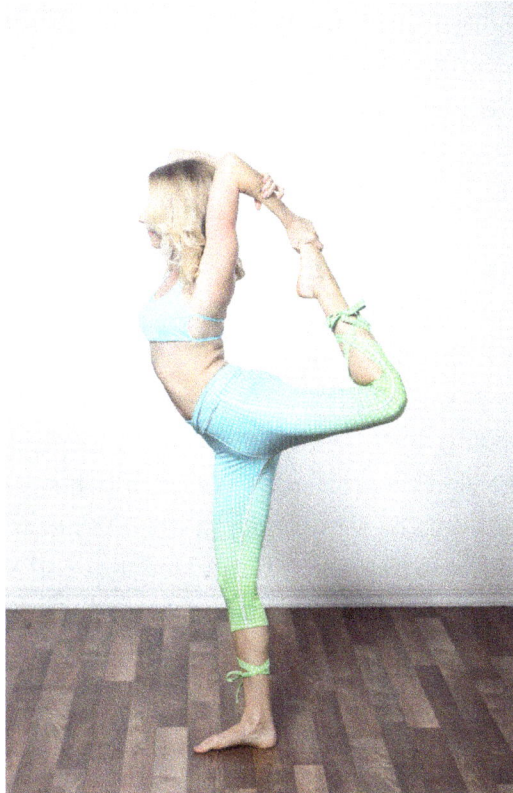

Knowing exercise is something we need to do is not always enough to motivate us to get up and move. Exercise is not really an option, but a non-negotiable part of life. Our bodies were designed to move! There are different reasons why people choose to exercise and some of those reasons include weight loss, fitness, stress management, physical therapy, or vanity goals. Some take it easy, and some go hard. It depends what your goals are. We are taught that exercise is a good thing for us, and, indeed, it is! I could sit here all day and preach to you about the importance of exercise, how to do it, and how it will keep you fit and fabulous. Yes, exercise does all that, but looking better is just a side effect. The quality of your life depends on you being physically active. You only have one life to live, so I encourage you to make exercise a daily part of your life to live it to the fullest.

As children, we were naturally active. We played tag outside with our friends and siblings, ran around during recess at school, and participated in sports or dance classes. We did not think to ourselves, "Gee, I better work out today." Life was much simpler back then. Children do not feel burdens in life quite like adults do. These burdens can make us feel uninspired to exercise due to long hours at work, parenting responsibilities, household chores, financial stress, relational stress, etc. The burdens and stressors are the reasons why exercise IS necessary. Exercise irons out troubles and clears the mind. As adults, we have freedom, giving us the ability to choose how we spend our time. If we indulge in over eating or drinking alcohol regularly, that inhibits our will to become a better version of ourselves.

To truly take care of our bodies and minds, we need to build self-discipline, meaning we participate in movement for our own good whether we feel like it or not. Once exercise becomes a habit after a month or two, you may find yourself addicted to it. After skipping a few days, you will miss the great overall feeling you are rewarded with from a good workout. Runners often become addicted to the activity of running and jogging due to the "runner's high" experienced from endorphins released in the brain. These feel-good brain chemicals provide a list of benefits that are too good to pass up and are essentially free natural drugs. By exercising, you will discover an improved self-image, better sleep quality, reduced stress, and enhanced moods. Frequent exercise also alleviates PMS symptoms, improves cardiovascular function, and builds muscle that boosts metabolism. In addition, you can beat off feelings of anxiety and depression with regular exercise.

You can see why exercise is so important for not only your body, but for your mind as well. Again, I challenge you to move every day! People often think they do not have the energy to work out. This is not necessarily true. The intensity of your daily exercise should vary based on your needs. You can always do something, whether it's an energy shifting yoga practice, a neighborhood walk, weight lifting/toning, a high intensity training burst, or a dance workout video. The key is to engage in something every day. There may be times of exhaustion when rest is necessary, and a twenty-minute nap or a ten-minute meditation just may give you what you need to feel refreshed enough to work out.

Of course, if you are ill, you should rest and recover. Listen to your body to help you determine what kind of workout is appropriate for you that day. When you give energy through movement, you get energy. This creates an instant state change. Feeling lethargic? Get up and jump up and down for a few minutes. You will feel enlivened. Not only will you be energized after a toning workout, but your muscles continue to work at burning fat and calories.

Throughout my life, I've always been involved in a sport, like soccer or baseball, or an extracurricular activity, like cheerleading, dance class, or my high school marching band. Near the end of my senior year of high school, my best friend and I decided we wanted to work out at a gym, probably because we wanted to look fit, toned, and cute. My desire to stay fit stuck with me after my freshman year of college when I gained fifteen pounds from reasons you can probably infer. I noticed that when I exercised, I had higher energy levels, and my blood pressure was quite good. I took weight training classes and lifting weights helped me reduce body fat and build lean muscle. My interest in fitness education also taught me that weight bearing exercise increases bone density. I became hooked!

From there, I became obsessed with ballet and yoga, taking any and every class I could get myself into both inside and out of college. Exercise naturally improves many things without the latest drug, pill, or quick fix. Find physical activities you enjoy doing so you are more likely to engage in them. Pair up with a friend, partner, or group for your favorite activities. This will make exercise more fun, and it will feel less like another chore to check off the list. Every single day, fit in thirty to sixty minutes of physical activity as this will optimize your life. I know it optimizes mine!

Nobody is completely motivated to work out all the time, so here are some tips for what to do when you really do not want to exercise. The most important thing to remember is, even when you have those resistant feelings, doing it anyway will leave you feeling happier than before. You will feel better afterwards, and if you recognize that ahead of time, you will be more empowered to just do it. Nike killed it with their slogan, "Just do it," because you really just have to do it and the positivity follows the action.

People who exercise regularly are happier, and parents who exercise set a good example for their family. Involve your children if possible. You can jog to the park and have your child (children) bike, scooter, or jog along with you. Here are some other ways to stay active and involve your children: Play your favorite songs and have yourselves a dance party. Get your boogie on in the living room and around the house. Park farther away from your destination in parking lots to get in more steps, or drive halfway there and make it a point to walk the rest of the way. House cleaning is a light physical activity, so if you're cleaning house, that counts. If the TV is on, make the commercial breaks fitness breaks for you and the kids. Have them help make up names for pushups, squats, and sit ups, like mermaid sit ups, Minnie Mouse squats, or Spider-Man pushups. Take turns being the coach by calling out moves or play Follow the Leader with impromptu jumps, moves, or wiggles. Try making your own "fit" deck of cards, each having an exercise pictured on it. Your kids may enjoy making them with you. Call it your "fitness project." In addition, you can walk the dog(s) or take a nature walk in the neighborhood to see how many animals you can spot, like birds, dogs, or cats. There are plenty of ways to incorporate physical activity into your daily routine, and it doesn't have to be overly strenuous. It is not necessary to pay memberships to gyms or boutique classes, although it's nice to visit those places from time to time to mix it up and keep the routine fresh. I love going to yoga, Pilates, spin, and dance classes myself. Most places will give you a free trial for your first visit! Take advantage of that and try something new.

Gyms and studios are great if the prices are within your budget and your schedule allows. Working with and being around other people is uplifting and can help us get our minds off worries. I used to work out in a gym for years, and then decided to work out at home due to time constraints. Working out at home and outdoors is just as effective, plus, you get sunshine, fresh air, and you save travel time and money. All you must do is make the time and space for yourself. Let your family know that your exercise time is important and cannot be interrupted. If you have an infant, nap, meditate, and exercise when the little angel is sleeping. Some of the pros about gyms are most of them have a variety of activities to offer all in one place, like tennis courts, swimming pools, saunas, steam rooms, cardio equipment, weight machines, free weights, group fitness classes, and sometimes child care. Gyms are also great places to meet other people who want to get in shape and stay fit.

It is up to you to figure out what is going to work best for your budget and schedule and stick with a plan. If you are lacking motivation, then change it up, try a new activity, and find something inspiring to motivate you. Think about how good you are going to feel and look afterwards. Variety is the spice of life, and there are so many ways to be active. Make a list of your favorite activities, like walking, jogging, running, or gardening. Do you love having a clean house? Blast your favorite tunes and clean away. Love the outdoors and sunshine? Try biking, swimming, yoga at the beach, hiking, or tennis. Love basketball? Find a group to play with on the regular. Pick what you would like to do or try and go for it. Set some fitness goals now. Start small if you must. Think, *Today, I will do ten minutes of cardio and ten minutes of stretching. Next week, and each consecutive week thereafter, I will add five minutes more cardio to my routine and continue to build from there.* Changing up your routine by varying your workouts keeps you engaged and helps avoid plateaus by keeping your body guessing. Lasting results come this way, because dreaded and arduous workout plans are like diets. You can suffer through them to the end, but afterwards, get over it and go back to something else, or completely fall off the wagon. If you do fall off the wagon, just get back on and build yourself back up. It's never too late.

Aim to work in thirty to sixty minutes a day of physical activity, four to five times a week. Even on the other few "off days," take a twenty-minute walk around the neighborhood after dinner while listening to your favorite songs or chatting with a partner. Try listening to an inspiring podcast to keep your mind focused on enrichment, growth, and self-development. If you are just getting started with an exercise routine and have any pre-existing health concerns, consult with your doctor to discuss what some good choices for you would be. Walking and yoga are great choices because they relieve stress and are not overly strenuous.

Why force yourself to engage in something you don't like? There are so many fabulous and affordable workout programs you can access online from your phone, tablet, or computer. Keeping your space clean and in order will allow for positive energy to flow at home and you will feel more inclined to work out there. Light a candle and use an aromatherapy diffuser. Essential oil scents used in aromatherapy diffusers are great for uplifting moods, relieving stress, and promoting relaxation. You don't need a ton of space to get a productive workout in. You can find great indoor workouts on YouTube, ranging from walking indoors to dance workouts, high intensity training, yoga, and Pilates. Take advantage of the different tools and resources available to help you along the way, ensuring that you have no excuse not to exercise.

In addition to the physiological benefits, exercise increases beauty! It creates a healthy glow—a look you can't buy from a bottle. There is only so much creams and facial products could accomplish on the outside. Exercise brings beauty from the inside out, detoxifies, oxygenates the cells, and assists in achieving tight, youthful, and beautiful skin. The quality of your life depends on it, and your beauty will increase.

CHAPTER 13
SLAYING GIANTS

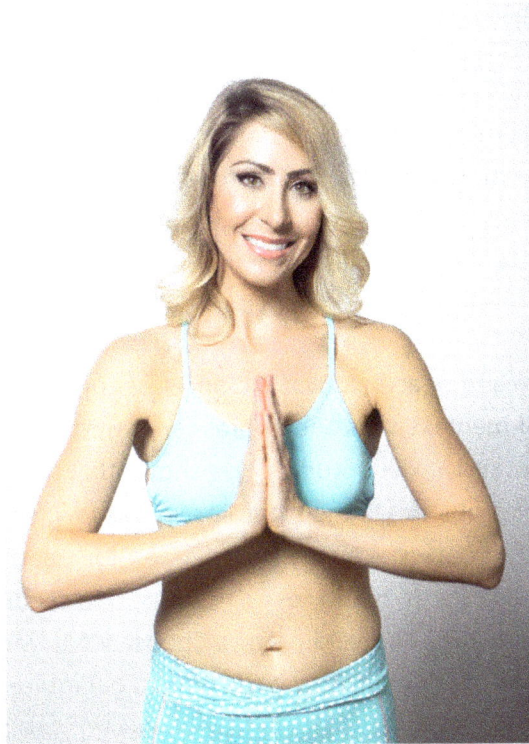

Food is one form of nourishment and we need it to survive. Food is a secondary form of nourishment, however, because other aspects in life feed us in important ways as well and I'll refer to them as primary foods. Primary foods are what feed our soul, and they all have important places in each of our lives. These aspects of life include relationships, love, connection, touch, fun, laughter, cheerfulness, work you love, spirituality, gratitude, giving, adventure, hobbies, financial stability, fresh air, and sunshine, to name a few. These parts of life essentially contribute to our health and happiness, your best self and, ultimately, your best life. Know that a happy and fulfilled life is yours for the taking. You must seek it and choose it. Stress, anxiety, depression, and mental health are integral aspects of wellbeing, and millions of people are affected by various experiences with these factors at different stages in life. According to the National Institute of Mental Health, 40 million Americans between the ages of 18-54 suffer from anxiety disorders.[103] Maintaining sound mental health is equally as important as diet and exercise for wellness.

Mental Health and Nutrition

The next question to ponder, analogous to the chicken and egg relationship, is which one must precede the other concerning health? Nutrition or mental health? They go hand-in-hand, with a synergistic relationship. Nutrition is the foundation for all else, and it contributes to a positive mentality, increased physical energy, and more confidence, which improves other areas in life, such as relationships. The mind is like a garden. It may become overtaken with negative thoughts like weeds. We must work to keep positive thoughts present in the mind like blooming flowers.

Having healthy skin and peace of mind are priceless components of health. Chronic stress over time puts one at risk for mental illness and depression. Nutritionally, there are ways to combat and manage acne, depression, and anxiety. Studies have shown that people who suffer from acne and depression have low levels of probiotics in their stool, as well as low levels of omega-3 fatty acids.[104] Eating foods with omega-3 fatty acids is also recommended for people with anxiety. Plant based sources of omega-3 include: flax seeds, hemp seeds, walnuts, chia seeds, microalgae oil, purslane (a green leafy vegetable), grape leaves, and wild berries. Choose what you eat wisely and if you have never considered the condition of your gut, now is the time to get interested.

A healthy gut microflora and probiotics can positively influence inflammation, glycemic control, mood, fat regulation, and acne. Prebiotics and probiotics are your new best friends. In a study involving forty-four patients with irritable bowel syndrome, the oral consumption of a prebiotic fiber combined with probiotics significantly reduced anxiety.[105]

Prebiotics are non-digestible foods that allow the growth of beneficial microorganisms in the intestines, and they work together with probiotics for a healthier intestinal environment. Some examples of prebiotic foods are those that are raw and high in fiber, such as chicory root, Jerusalem ar-

---

103   Anxiety and Depression Association of America. (2010-2016) Facts and Statistics. Retrieved from https://adaa.org/about-adaa/press-room/facts-statistics#

104   Bowe, Whitney P, and Alan C Logan. "Acne Vulgaris, Probiotics and the Gut-Brain-Skin Axis - back to the Future?" *Gut Pathogens 3* (2011): 1. PMC. Web. 18 Apr. 2017.

105   Bowe, Whitney P, and Alan C Logan. "Acne Vulgaris, Probiotics and the Gut-Brain-Skin Axis - back to the Future?" Gut Pathogens 3 (2011): 1. PMC. Web. 3 Apr. 2017.

tichoke, dandelion greens, garlic, leeks, onion, asparagus, and banana. Cooking these foods will lessen the prebiotic properties and reduce their enzymatic properties. Eating them raw is important because you will get the most benefits from the prebiotics and the most energy and rejuvenating properties from the foods. You can add fresh garlic to salad dressings, guacamole, pâtés, and hummus. Eating fresh parsley will help neutralize the garlic smell.

Avoid processed sugar because it feeds yeast, which eats away at the intestinal wall and crowds out good bacteria. We need good bacteria in our gut to fight disease for a strong immune system and healthy digestion. This may seem overwhelming to some people, but the truth is, when you adopt a truly healthy lifestyle, all those issues tend to take care of themselves. The key is to know how to bring yourself into balance naturally because the body was designed to do this.

We must be conscious about how the primary foods in our lives are affecting us, and when one is out of balance. You could eat the purest and cleanest daily diet, keeping your body and mind physiologically functioning—foundational for great health and beauty. On the other hand, if you are struggling with finances, feeling unfulfilled in your career, have a lack of spirituality, or are in toxic relationships, these things are adverse to your health. You could still be unhealthy due to those things despite eating the healthiest diet on the planet. Begin by loving and accepting yourself, forgiving yourself and others, practicing gratitude, and helping others through giving. You deserve to be happy and fulfilled. Your feelings matter.

Stress affects our mentality, physiology, relationships, and can lead to depression. We must start by building an awareness of what stresses us out, making conscious decisions, moment by moment, to not let stress consume our happiness or health. This is what I call slaying the giants in our lives. How about we don't give into letting stress win and choose to control it by having a plan for how we will respond when stressors arise? Sure, we all fall down. Sometimes, we fall hard, and life may seem hopeless. I fall, too. The key is to get back up and remember there is always hope for a better tomorrow. Interactions with others, thought patterns, and emotional intelligence affects your health. Identify where your sources of stress are coming from. Do you put too much on your plate? Do you allow toxic relationships to drag you down? If so, it's time to set boundaries around those people and situations. Communicate with others about your needs, and if you are not respected, love yourself enough to keep distance from that which is not serving you. Know your limits and don't demand so much of yourself that you don't have any time to relax or have fun. Having unstructured downtime is essential for everyone.

Stress is quite a buzzword in society, and we latch onto it like it's some sort of parasite that's worked its way into our lives. I challenge you to turn your stress into passion as you work towards the dreams that matter to you. If you are unhappy in one area, take some time to focus on what you need to do to make a change. Don't listen to the voices telling you that you can't do it or you're not good enough. Nothing can stress you out or upset you unless you let it. This is easier said than done. I am still working on this one. It just takes some practice and boundary setting to get yourself to a place of truth and recognition.

People are imperfect and will let you down from time to time. Usually, the ill feelings we experience come from our mindset about a situation. We need to learn how to think, control our emotions, and not react to negative triggers in life. Learn what your triggers are and devise a plan of action for how you will deal with them when they arise. Surround yourself with positive people who support you. We were all created to experience peace, joy, and love. Be a bringer of happiness and excitement to life, even when it's hard.

Acceptance is another great lesson to learn and practice. Accept what you cannot change and respond strategically to what you can change by acting towards your goals. Though life is hard at times, we can still smile, shine, and love through the pain. Our experiences and ability to overcome difficulties in life allows us to help others going through similar situations. One way to create awareness around this is to list three of your greatest challenges or current life triggers in a journal. They could be people, situations, negative thoughts, or feelings. Once you list the triggers, list how you are going to deal with each one in a healthy way as they arise. This practice is powerful and gives you strength. If you don't have journal, I recommend getting one to keep on hand to write in as often as possible.

Nobody is immune from life stressors. It's really a matter of when the negativity will rise and attack you. Be ready to defeat it. Stress management action plans include self-care, setting boundaries, daily prayer/meditation, healthy communication, breathwork, pure food, and exercise. Work these things into your week regularly and you will feel and see a difference. Things that once stressed you out a lot may shrink down into nothingness. Even if the things stressing you out are important, not reacting to the stress does not mean you don't care. It just means you can process life situations in a way that is better for you and those around you.

Complacency does nothing, and we want to move forward towards our purpose and destiny. You are meant for amazing things in alignment with your gifts and talents. Everybody is gifted in different ways and has an important purpose on this earth. We all get down sometimes, but the trick is not to stay down. When you feel low, recognize it. Allow yourself time to mourn for what's mourn-worthy. Take the initiative to beat it in that moment by changing your state with exercise and breathing techniques. Like a champion, we must get back up, dust off, and never quit this thing called life. Each day, we have a chance to become better versions of ourselves. Controlling anxiety and depression without medication is possible with an open mind, will, and determination. If your issues are extreme, consult your doctor and/or seek therapy/psychotherapy, or phone a close friend or family member. Do not be too proud to reach out for help. We all need to do that from time to time.

A lot of people are prescribed medication to help them alleviate symptoms of depression and anxiety. It's important to know the implications of taking medicine for these things. Common side effects are insomnia, sexual dysfunction, upset stomach, headaches, increase in blood pressure, constipation, and blurred vision, just to name a few. Medications can be effective for people with chronic cases, but not so much for people with mild cases. Alternative treatments can be just as effective, if not more so, without the nasty side effects. These treatments include relaxation techniques, meditation, yoga, massage, acupuncture, and deep breathing. Stress sends the whole body into a whirlwind of dysfunction, and the immune system becomes compromised over time with chronic stress.[106]

Stress, anxiety, and depression are three words that stand alone, and three words that are often interwoven. When somebody feels anxiety, it leads to stress, and this prolonged over time leads to depression. It feels like you are walking down a dark tunnel searching for the end, to see the light, but it's not in sight. Stress is something we all experience from time to time depending on the work we do and our goals in life. It comes extrinsically from areas like family matters, parenting, the pursuit of higher education, finances, job relations, or self-created stress. Let's face it. Sometimes, we make mountains out of molehills, we stand in our own way, and our worries don't ever manifest themselves after all. American culture is fast paced, and we often pick up on messages from the world that more is better, bigger is better, and the grass is greener on the other side. This leaves us feeling empty or void, wrapped up in consumerist materialism. The grass is greener where you water it, and peace doesn't come from things outside of us.

I find that inner peace comes from a connectedness with God, trusting that my life is in the hands of something greater than myself for the good of all. The reality is we cannot control what happens to us in life, we can only control how we react. Mindfulness and meditation is helpful for creating peace of mind as well as letting go of things that don't serve you. Being in nature is another

---

106   Segerstrom, Suzanne C., and Gregory E. Miller. "Psychological Stress and the Human Immune System: A Meta-Analytic Study of 30 Years of Inquiry." *Psychological bulletin* 130.4 (2004): 601–630. PMC. Web. 5 Aug. 2017.

way to relax and find inner peace. Some people tend to over analyze, make up stories in their minds, and care too much about what people think about them. Fear of being judged can make us feel as if we shouldn't do things like be ourselves, speak up, act, or express our gifts and talents. Anxiety and fear make us feel as if something bad might happen as a result and that is not true. People probably don't care as much as you think they do, and if they want to judge you, let them. Who cares anyway?

The daily grind can weigh you down, contributing to unwanted feelings of unhappiness. As women, expectations tend to fall on our shoulders to keep house, look amazing, raise children, work, and do many other things under the sun. It's not healthy to bear the pressure of having it all and doing it all. It can become quite cumbersome to keep up with life's responsibilities. Learning how to say *no* is a life changer! You don't have to be everything to everybody. When stress bites and we have reached our breaking point, it can have negative effects on our health and relationships. This hinders our ability to be loving, nurturing, and the truly amazing people we are. How many times have I buckled under the pressures of trying to keep up with being the ideal 21st century woman? You mindlessly snap at your children, go off on a friend, or push away a loved one. You may be wondering, *Who is this person?* You know what I'm talking about, ladies. It means your needs are not being met in some way. Either you need love, space, relaxation, or a slower pace. This is where we need to give ourselves a time out to reflect, step back, and then react intentionally.

Knowing how to deal with stress through understanding its root cause and keeping it in check will allow you to be in control of your life and emotions. I am not saying that it will be easy, but stress management will improve the quality of your life, allowing you to live more fully aware and present in the moment. Begin by declaring this right now to yourself: "I will not allow anything or anyone to ultimately steal the peace and joy I deserve in life." Choose and embrace this idea. By doing so, we are not denying negative emotions. I don't recommend that. We create an awareness and acknowledgement of them. If we stop to feel and accept them, we can learn to pause and breathe through them. This allows us to control our triggers with emotional intelligence. It's not like we ever reach a destination of perfection. Instead, we are a work in progress. We must face the mountains in our lives, moving them little by little, one day at a time. Arm yourself with knowledge and tools for how to deal with negativity when the fear, anger, and frustration pour down like acid rain. Take a step back when you are feeling overwhelmed and ask yourself if your problem is as big as you are making it out to be. Then, approach it from a solution standpoint instead of a reactive standpoint.

When slaying the giants in our lives, every beauty queen needs to armor herself with rest.

Sleep contributes to health immensely, and I had to learn that for myself the hard way. For a lot of things, "less is more," but not when it comes to sleep. I used to skimp on sleep to work, socialize, or worry, and that is downright dangerous. I now take sleep seriously and have made it a priority by coming up with a nighttime routine. Our bodies are restored during sleep, and not properly sleeping deteriorates the brain's ability to think and the body's ability to function. Less than six hours is not ideal, and seven to nine hours is golden. When I sleep enough, it feels as if I can deal with whatever life throws at me much better than if I slept less than seven hours. In cases when I sleep four to five hours, I am about as good as a bull in a china closet at my daily performance.

When sleep is deficient, thinking is impaired, and making good decisions becomes difficult. I'm also much more emotional when I don't sleep enough. A couple of times, I skipped a night of sleep due to business travel and having to work the next day. My brain was literally flatlined and I was as spacey as ever, like an alien from another planet. Completely zoned out, I was merely breathing those few days, quite good for nothing. I could barely think or put a sentence together. Imagine the turmoil a persistent reduced sleep habit can cause a person. A lack of sleep has been linked to depression, risky behavior, suicide, obesity, heart disease, kidney disease, and high blood pressure.[107] When you are sleep deprived, your body makes less leptin (a hormone that makes you feel full) and makes more ghrelin (the hormone that makes you want to eat more). Let's not forget that a good night's rest makes you look better, too! The phrase "beauty sleep" has merit. The haggard, sleepless look doesn't fair well on anybody and contributes to wrinkles and under eye bags. I don't care how much eye cream and concealer you use. Those products cannot do for you what sleep does. Sleep increases blood flow to the face and makes you look younger. Are you ready to start taking your sleep seriously?

Sleeping less, eating poorly, drinking a lot of alcohol, smoking, and failure to exercise are ingredients for a recipe of disaster. If you allow yourself to be worried and anxious all the time, work yourself to the bone without time to rest and relax, you are bound to burn out in a major way or have a nervous breakdown. American culture embraces the "grind" and hustle of working hard and playing hard, and the idea of doing nothing is looked down upon as being lazy. There is nothing wrong with the hustle, however, you must know where to draw the line, differentiating a healthy hustle versus a debilitating grind. Health = life! Time for rest and relaxation is necessary for everyone, and I recommend you schedule it into your week.

How you feel when you do "nothing?" For many of us, doing nothing is a rare moment, and it's hard to do just that if you are a type A, highly driven individual. It's hard for me. Type A personali-

---

107   https://www.nhlbi.nih.gov/health/health-topics/topics/sdd/why

ties are competitive, impatient, aggressive, outgoing, ambitious, and perfectionistic. My fellow type A readers: it's okay, you are not alone, and life can be difficult sometimes because people generally do not respond well nor understand the drive we feel inside. On the other hand, type B personalities are more relaxed and easy going. You may find yourself to have both personalities at times. We all must channel the type B in us from time to time. Balance is the goal. Here is a word of caution to all my type A friends and angry birds: You are predisposed to stress because you are driven and hardcore. Be mindful of your tendencies and learn to manage your triggers. You could have a plan for this and, in doing so, would be doing yourself and your relationships a favor. Life will be so much sweeter. The art of doing nothing is something to indulge in from time to time to allow yourself adequate time to recharge. One day a week is a good amount of time to unplug from the grind, email, social media, and life's demands. Keep a daily planner and schedule in all the things you need to get done for the week in six days. Then clear one day to rest, relax, and recharge. Do something that truly fills you up in alignment with your gifts and talents, like take a dance class or play a group sport. Do not be afraid to turn down an invitation or event you feel obligated to attend, but truly don't want to. If you are feeling particularly off balance, frazzled, exhausted, overworked, out of sorts, unhappy, or just plain stressed out, ask yourself what you need. Take some time to breathe, meditate and pray, asking for guidance and clarity.

By connecting with your feelings and needs, you are better able to take care of yourself, and this allows you to better take care of others. You will never regret taking time for yourself, and by doing this, you will improve the relationships in your life, including the one you have with yourself. People snap, bark, and break because their cup isn't full, meaning they are missing out on what they need. For example, getting a massage after work when you're feeling stressed will send you home relaxed and refreshed. A good massage can wipe away a bad day, let alone a bad week. Rather than going home frazzled, grumpy, and ready to eat a half gallon of ice cream, you can address your needs in a self-loving way. Take a hot bath and go to bed early instead of drinking alcohol to cope. A hot bath, deep breathing, and a good book is a much better idea and less debilitating.

When anxiety strikes, in the case of a panic attack, it can feel like walls are closing in, and physical symptoms might arise. These types of attacks have happened to me before and it feels like chest pain, dizziness, fear, helplessness, sweating, weakness, stomach pain, numbness/tingling, or a pounding, racing heart, fatigue, insomnia, and headaches. It's a horrible feeling that sometimes comes out of nowhere. Let's say you are truly dissatisfied with your job, feeling apprehension or dread about going there, and you have trouble concentrating throughout the day. This dread leaves you feeling irritable, with uncontrollable, intrusive thoughts that taunt your mind. I know this is true be-cause I have felt and been through all of it. If you feel like you have a panic or stress disorder, seek help and talk to your doctor. Sometimes these symptoms might be caused by a medical condition such as asthma, hypoglycemia, or a thyroid problem.

I started getting panic attacks when I was seventeen, out of the blue, for no apparent rea-son. I remember this happened to me when I was in a Lake Tahoe casino with a friend. An attack came out of nowhere and I had to go back to the cabin right away to hide out with a bellowing migraine that sent me straight to a dark room with a bed and plenty of Advil until the episode subsided.

Being able to manage stress is at the cornerstone of our health and survival. Here are some simple strategies to use when dealing with mild to moderate anxiety, stress, and depression. Take some time for yourself whether it's listening to music, practicing yoga, or journaling. Doing one or many of these activities helps distance yourself from your worries and fears. Studies have shown that relaxation and physiological benefits gained from practicing yoga relieves high blood pressure and assists in relieving arthritis, arteriosclerosis, chronic fatigue, asthma, and varicose veins. One study on the effects of a regular and ongoing yoga practice revealed reduced body weight, increased lung capacity, improved stress resistance, and a decrease in blood sugar levels and cholesterol. Stress man-agement is preventative and restorative medicine.

Make sure to eat well balanced plant-based meals high in raw fruits and vegetables. Limit caffeine and alcohol consumption since they trigger panic attacks and heighten anxiety, and choose to drink water and herbal teas instead. Try making your own fruit infused water at home by soaking fruit like cucumbers, strawberries, lemon, and herbs like mint in water to give it delicious flavor. When you are feeling tense, frustrated or angry, count to ten slowly, take deep breaths by inhaling and ex-haling slowly with one hand on your heart and one hand on your belly. Do not overload or pressure yourself too much with anything.

One way to ground yourself when feeling overwhelmed, stressed, or anxious is to breathe. This sounds like stating the obvious because it's something you do anyway. What I am referring to here is deep breathing exercises. Deep breathing can do a lot to revolutionize your health. It was the missing link to my wellness routine for a long time. Once I started incorporating breathwork, my health improved, and I could control my anxiety and better oversee my emotions. Here is a breath routine you can use throughout the day as needed to soothe and relax your mind and body: Take a long, slow deep breath in for four counts, hold it for four counts, and exhale for four counts. Repeat this four times for an instant calming effect.

Remember to do your best rather than trying to be perfect all the time. Accept and love yourself no matter how well you perform. Ask yourself if the situation is as bad as you think by putting it into perspective. Practice having a positive attitude by replacing negative thoughts with positive thoughts and gratitude for the blessings you have in life. Give back to your community by volunteering or plugging into a support network that takes your mind off yourself and your stressors. Like I've said before, no matter who you are, there are times in life when you may fall into a rut. Life happens, and people face times of loneliness, endure grief, battle depression, loss, or emotional turmoil due to various factors. These things, whether self-induced or not, downright stop us in our tracks. In dealing with those things, recognizing there is always hope is the first step to making it through. Getting out into new surroundings and doing something different really helps.

Mundane activities in life can become drudgery. When you are feeling low and worthless, I understand that doing anything feels like an unwanted chore. Feelings of worthlessness are liars! Those feelings make you feel like you aren't good enough, smart enough, or talented enough. They ask, "Who are you to have that success, be beautiful, or get the job?" Fight them! Focus on what you do want to happen with faith and envision it. Sometimes, we make up nightmarish outcomes in our own minds that haven't even happened nor will they ever happen. If somebody says something to you out of fear or confusion and you let it upset you, it might send you into a downward spiral. Negative thinking can also lead us down a depressed and saddened road, wasting our precious energy on nothingness with roused up emotions. Has that ever happened to you? You get all worked up and upset about something, perhaps made up some scenarios or entertained some negative (but untrue) thoughts in your head, and then the situation worked itself out in the end, and the emotional stress and feelings of unhappiness were unnecessary. Trusting the process in life and being mindful of the silver lining in store is good to remember. Shake up your schedule if possible and do things in a different order. Talk to new people, smile at them, or strike up conversation. Becoming hyper focused on ourselves and problems causes us to lose joy. Mind control is an important part of mental health, which affects other areas of health. Learn how to control your mind and manage your emotions. You will be happier and more successful in this game of life.

How many of you are unhappy with your job? Like, really unhappy? How would it feel to devise a plan and take action on an exit strategy to leave that job situation and step into one that is rewarding and energizing? Step away from that relationship, distance yourself from negative people, or whatever it is that brings you down. You must not let people who don't accept or love you uncondi-tionally discourage you in life. These people may be those you love, family members, or even yourself. It's okay to love them anyway, but you are not bound to be around negativity. Never stop looking for a way out of a toxic situation because the answer is out there. Even during chaos, there is light at the end of the tunnel.

CHAPTER 14
NOW IS YOUR TIME TO SHINE

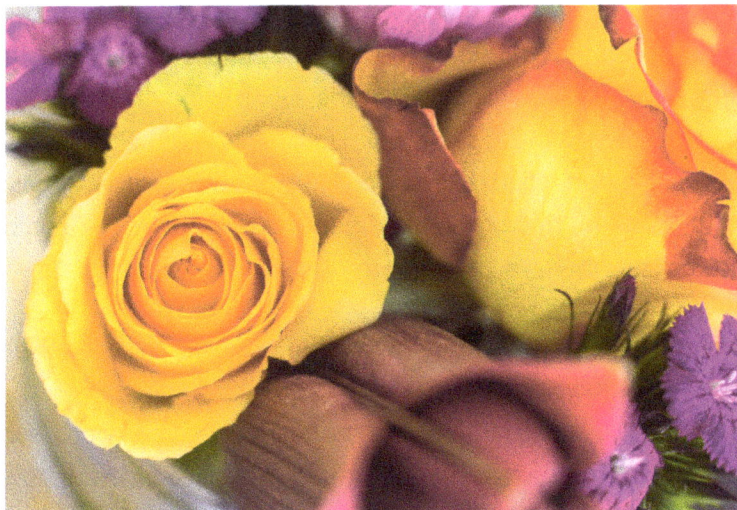

~ Become all you are meant to be ~

We are our own worst critics. Being confident is something that many people struggle with. Your confidence will increase the more you exercise your confidence muscles. By this, I do not mean working your biceps or hamstrings. Practicing the act of being confident and believing in yourself will make you feel more confident. Even if you do not feel confident, act like you are and face that fear. No one else knows how you feel inside and what you are thinking. Guess what will happen once you choose confidence, self-acceptance, and start loving yourself and who you are? The rest of the world will see that, and you will begin to attract more of what you what you want in your life. We are all born to make a difference in this world, no matter how big or how small. I challenge you to be empowered and tap into that divine connection leading you to your destiny. The idea that we can create our lives through choice is truth. We are like painters and life is the canvas. Having the choice to paint it beauti-fully is a gift, no matter where you begin. Exceptional paintings take a great deal of time to complete.

Look at your life this way: You are the artist working on the details of the painting of your life day by day, year after year, executing every brushstroke. You are a beautiful work of art and are always a work in progress. No matter how much we grow, each day is an opportunity for improvement, and like wine, we can allow ourselves to get better with age. If we are growing, changing, and evolving, we are constantly learning and climbing higher, unless we settle for less.

In college, I majored in Art Studio, and would spend hours in the studio with my paint, brushes, and canvas. If I made a mistake, I could reshape, refine, or paint over the line or brushstroke to make it appear the way I intended. In the same way, life has a way of being shaped if we, as the artist, live with intention. Life is not perfect, and we are not meant to be perfect either. Our mistakes work themselves out, and through the mistakes and smoothing over the rough patches, we can emerge with strength and power. Our story can inspire and encourage someone else at some point.

Failure is only a learning opportunity, and the most successful people in the world are said to have failed forward with perseverance, and this is the quintessential trait of success. Know that you are okay, and all is well. It takes belief, faith, divine connection, and an open heart with the ability to stay connected to one's own true self; staying grounded in a place of peace, love, forgiveness, generosity, and surrendering to thrive and live your life out loud. Let go of fears, whatever yours are, and make a list of everything you want to achieve and experience in your life, no matter how lofty the goals may be. There is power in thinking big, and why not do this for yourself? Imagine if Walt Disney put a ceiling on his imaginative ideas and gave up on his dreams. This man overcame many obstacles including financial destitution and verbal attacks against his talents. He had to beg an investor friend for six years just to get the Disneyland Hotel funded and built. Beginning as a farm boy in the country, he is now a legend and his legacy will live on forever. When Walt was getting started as an animator, he was broke, desperate, found himself homeless, and could not pay his animation team. Yet he persevered and eventually became successful after years of angst and struggle. I am so glad he didn't quit, and you should not give up on yourself and your dreams either. Who cares how old you are or what other people think about your pursuits. We have one life to live and what are you living it for?

Think big right now and take out your journal. Write a list of everything you wish to achieve physically, mentally, spiritually, career related, and financially. What kind of lifestyle would you like? Do you want to be lean, full of energy, debt-free, calm, mentally stable, and living with passion? Are you working to bring in money doing work in alignment with your talents, and are you giving back in a way that contributes to a greater cause than yourself? This embodies greatness. Make that goals list right now, and next to each list, give a timeline of when you would like to have achieved those goals, anywhere from right now, this year, to three years, five years, ten years, and twenty years from now. How would you like to live in terms of truth, health, fitness, creativity, and spirituality? Do you need to think outside the box to experience freedom and a judgement-free perspective? What does freedom mean to you? Is it living pain-free, without a dependence on medication? Is it being able to work for yourself in your bathrobe or running a meaningful business that helps others as well? We must make our decisions in alignment with what we want for the future, and not miss out on the joy of the moment, which is all we really have. Tomorrow will always be a day we chase. Note that joy and happiness are different. Being happy is an emotion and it's fleeting. We aren't always going to feel happy, but joy is more of a choice—something we can embrace through the varying emotions we experience in life when things do or don't work out our way, because they won't always.

The foundation to all which we experience in life begins with the health of our minds and bodies. Without those things, what can we do? What do we have? If we are sick, overweight, dependent on medication, lack confidence and energy then we are merely living, not thriving. The opposite is available to us: energy, peace, rest, health, vibrancy, and love. All of the money in the world cannot buy you health, love, or happiness. We must attract what we want by knowing what it is and by not doubting ourselves. Feel and imagine it as if it is happening, envision what you want every day, be grateful and thankful for what you do have going on for yourself, and trust the process of the journey. This is called faith and is when you are certain of what you wish for but do not see. Think of where you were a year ago, five years ago, or ten years ago. How has your life changed or improved over time? Did it go by fast? Look at what you overcame, and don't you feel stronger because of that? What did you learn, and where are you going in the next ten years? The key is to enjoy the journey, accepting that even though we may not have yet accomplished our goals, they might take time, or we may fail multiple times until we succeed.

Engage in learning. It's said that if you are not learning, you are dying. This makes life interesting and juicy, giving us much to look forward to. Do not limit yourself because of some limiting belief (like you're not pretty or smart enough). Sometimes these thoughts come out of nowhere, like the devil on your shoulder trying to scare you and get you down. Don't listen! Recognize that those thoughts are lies and tell yourself you are worthy, smart, and beautiful! It's never too late to get well, heal, lose fat, exercise, be in the best shape of your life, attain a meaningful career, engage in your favorite hobby, take a trip, sing, or dance. There are so many factors in life that are out of our control, and sometimes we mess up, but those setbacks never spell the end.

Gratitude and empowerment are cornerstones for a life well lived. Here are three questions to ask yourself every day for staying empowered and grateful. Go ahead and take a second to reflect and write them down now. Ready? Okay! One: what are you grateful for? Write down five things you are grateful for daily in a journal, or as often as possible to keep your mind and mentality in the right place. The second question you could ask yourself is: what makes me happy? If I'm not happy, what can I do to improve my life and get myself into a positive state? Finally, ask yourself: what can I do to be more giving, to make this world a better place? Look in the mirror and say to yourself with intent, "I am choosing to have peace today no matter what happens, even when things do not go my way." We cannot control the world, but we are in control of our thoughts and actions, which shape our feelings. It might feel exhausting to maintain positive thoughts all the time, so in being mindful, recognize your negative emotions and thoughts and choose not to act on them. Ignoring the negativity or putting on a front causes you to bottle up your emotions, and might be responsible for anger, which you might take out on others. It's key to find ways to channel that energy and not bottle it inside.

When I was going through hard times, I would put on a happy face to the world and bottle up all the negative things going on inside. Eventually, I would hit a wall and that's when the "bitch" would come out. It's important to realize that when people become prickly, it's for a reason. Try not to judge them, rather put yourself in their shoes and have empathy. This is yet another great lesson I learned that has changed my life. Keeping your actions and thoughts in check could revolutionize the way you live and will help you paint a beautiful picture of your life to look back on in the end.

A spiritual man once discussed the idea of attending your own funeral. "What did you contribute to this world, what impact did you make, and how did you live?" he asked. As he shared these questions, my soul began to shake. This made me realize that we never know when our last day will be, therefore, we must live each day to the fullest, giving the best of ourselves. How would we treat others and what would we do if it were our last day? Remembering this opens my heart, allows me to face fear, be more generous, relax, and accept what is. It helps me to slow down, step out, and share what needs to be said. I tell my daughter all the time how much I love her, and I say sorry when I'm wrong. It's quite liberating to be humble and to relish in the concept of being kind and giving (even when you don't feel like it). This concept is so powerful to me, and it allows me to love the unlovable, pursue my dreams, endure life with grace, push through fatigue, and forgive the people who have wronged me. This all sounds so perfect doesn't it? I am certainly not, but life is about the journey, not the destination.

FINAL THOUGHTS

The world of nutrition and science can be dizzying with debating opinions on what is healthy versus what is not. We hear a lot of, "Eat this, not that!" *Beautiful Awakening* promotes a plant-based lifestyle for the greater good of all. I do this with hopes to inspire, improve, and save lives. Nobody is perfect, and we all have struggles, no matter how perfect our life appears to be on the outside. Many women and men struggle with eating disorders, hormonal imbalance, acne, poor digestion, low self-esteem, depression, anxiety, and more. These things could be overcome. I envision building a community of health warriors who support and encourage one another to be their best and give their best, stemming from a foundation of gratitude. We must learn to love ourselves, let go of negativity, and love one another despite our differences. After all, that is what life is all about.

ABOUT THE AUTHOR

Shelli Belleci grew up in California and lived there for most of her life. She enjoys art, makeup, singing, and dancing. Having an affinity for exercise and nutrition from a young age, she has worked through her own health challenges, which led her down a holistic path to healing. She has worked as a professional educator since 2005. After becoming certified as a health coach, Shelli envisioned Your Sweet Life, a practice to assist people in achieving their best selves by addressing the root causes of problems. Shelli specializes in plant-based nutrition with an emphasis on raw foods and lifestyle optimization. Her hopes are to help people live more impactful lives by first helping them to feel more alive, living in alignment with their true selves. She knows that as we become happier and healthier, the people around us are positively affected and the world becomes a better place.

INDEX

www.ingramcontent.com/pod-product-compliance
Lightning Source LLC
Chambersburg PA
CBHW080358030426
42334CB00024B/2921